Cardiac Imaging Cases

Cardiac Imaging Cases

Charles S. White, MD

Professor of Radiology and Medicine
Chief of Thoracic Radiology
Department of Diagnostic Radiology
University of Maryland Medical Center
Baltimore, Maryland

Joseph Jen-Sho Chen, MD

Cardiothoracic Fellow
Department of Diagnostic Radiology
University of Maryland Medical Center
Baltimore, Maryland

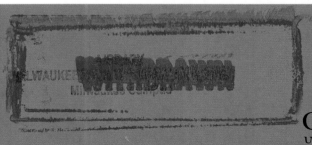

OXFORD
UNIVERSITY PRESS
2011

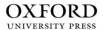

Oxford University Press, Inc., publishes works that further
Oxford University's objective of excellence
in research, scholarship, and education.

Oxford New York
Auckland Cape Town Dar es Salaam Hong Kong Karachi
Kuala Lumpur Madrid Melbourne Mexico City Nairobi
New Delhi Shanghai Taipei Toronto

With offices in
Argentina Austria Brazil Chile Czech Republic France Greece
Guatemala Hungary Italy Japan Poland Portugal Singapore
South Korea Switzerland Thailand Turkey Ukraine Vietnam

Published by Oxford University Press, Inc.
198 Madison Avenue, New York, New York 10016
www.oup.com

Oxford is a registered trademark of Oxford University Press.

Library of Congress Cataloging-in-Publication Data

White, Charles S.
Cardiac imaging cases / Charles S. White, Joseph Jen-Sho Chen.
p. ; cm.—(Cases in radiology)
Includes bibliographical references and indexes.
ISBN 978-0-19-539543-3
1. Heart—Imaging—Case Reports.   I. Chen, Joseph Jen-Sho.   II. Title.   III. Series: Cases in radiology.
[DNLM: 1. Diagnostic Imaging—Case Reports.   2. Heart Diseases—diagnosis—Case Reports.
WG 141 W583c 2011]
RC683.5.I42W55 2011
616.1'0754—dc22
2010013244

This material is not intended to be, and should not be considered, a substitute for medical or other professional advice. Treatment for the conditions described in this material is highly dependent on the individual circumstances. And, while this material is designed to offer accurate information with respect to the subject matter covered and to be current as of the time it was written, research and knowledge about medical and health issues is constantly evolving and dose schedules for medications are being revised continually, with new side effects recognized and accounted for regularly. Readers must therefore always check the product information and clinical procedures with the most up-to-date published product information and data sheets provided by the manufacturers and the most recent codes of conduct and safety regulation. The publisher and the authors make no representations or warranties to readers, express or implied, as to the accuracy or completeness of this material. Without limiting the foregoing, the publisher and the authors make no representations or warranties as to the accuracy or efficacy of the drug dosages mentioned in the material. The authors and the publisher do not accept, and expressly disclaim, any responsibility for any liability, loss or risk that may be claimed or incurred as a consequence of the use and/or application of any of the contents of this material.

9 8 7 6 5 4 3 2 1
Printed in China
on acid-free paper

To my wife, Ellen, for her steadfast support
in putting up with all the twists and turns that
an academic career entails. **C.S.W.**

To my wife, Eunju, for her patience,
support, and love. **J.J.C.**

Preface

This book provides an overview of cardiac imaging across the spectrum of cardiac disease. It is presented in an easy-to-read case-based format that includes the most recent information on each of these entities. Although the book is not intended to be comprehensive, wherever possible we have chosen classic images and distilled the most relevant information for those interested in learning cardiac imaging.

The book is divided into several parts. The first part consists of a brief review of basic anatomy. Subsequent parts are divided by disease category. Cases within each part have been placed in random order.

Although no book is all-inclusive, we hope this volume will assist you in your journey to master cardiac imaging.

Charles S. White, MD
Joseph Jen-Sho Chen, MD

Acknowledgments

We thank all of those who contributed to or assisted in obtaining some of the cases, particularly Dr. Jean Jeudy, M.D., of the University of Maryland (Cases 64, Cardiac Amyloidosis; 65, Cardiac Sarcoidosis; 66, Arrythmogenic Right Ventricular Dysplasia; and 68, Takotsubo Cardiomyopathy), Dr. Laura E. Heyneman, M.D., of Duke University (Case 56, Ventricular Septal Rupture), Dr. Jeffrey S. Mueller, M.D., of Allegheny General Hospital (Case 15, Cor Triatrium), and Dr. Jacob Kirsch, MD, of Cleveland Clinics (Case 11, Bland-White-Garland Syndrome).

The Publisher thanks the following for their time and advice:

Mark Anderson, University of Virginia
Sanjeev Bhalla, Mallinckrodt Institute of Radiology, Washington University
Michael Bruno, Penn State Hershey Medical Center
Melissa Rosado de Christenson, St. Luke's Hospital of Kansas City
Rihan Khan, University of Arizona
Angela Levy, Georgetown University
Alexander Mamourian, University of Pennsylvania
Stacy Smith, Brigham and Women's Hospital

Contents

Abbreviations

AA	amyloid associated
ACE	angiotensin converting enzyme
AcuteMarg	acute marginal
AICD	automated implantable cardioverter-defibrillator
aka	also known as
AL	amyloid light
ARVC	arrhythmogenic right ventricular cardiomyopathy
ARVD	arrhythmogenic right ventricular dysplasia
ASD	atrial septal defect
ATTR	amyloid Transthyretin
AV	atrioventricular
CABG	coronary artery bypass graft
CAC	coronary artery calcification
CCA	common carotid artery
CAD	coronary artery disease
CE	contrast enhancement
CECT	contrast-enhanced computed tomography
CHD	congestive heart disease
CHF	congestive heart failure
CM	cardiomyopathy
COPD	chronic obstructive pulmonary disease
CT	computed tomography
CTA	computed tomographic angiography
CT/MR	computed tomography/magnetic resonance
CXR	chest x-ray
CVA	cardiovascular accident
DM	diabetes mellitus
EBCT	electron beam computed tomography
ECG	electrocardiogram
ECHO	extracorporeal membrane oxygenation
EF	ejection fraction
FPP	first-pass perfusion
FS	fat saturation
GI	gastrointestinal

HIV	human immunodeficiency virus
HOCM	hypertrophic obstructive cardiomyopathy
HRCT	high-resolution computed tomography
HTN	hypertension
IACB	intra-aortic counterpulsion balloon
ICD	implantable cardioverter-defibrillator
IHSS	idiopathic hypertrophic subaortic stenosis
IMA	internal mammary artery
IPF	interstitial pulmonary fibrosis
IVC	inferior vena cava
LA	left atrium
LAD	left anterior descending
LBBB	left bundle branch block
LCA	left coronary artery
LCx	left circumflex
LLL	left lower lobe
LM	left main
LUL	left upper lobe
LV	left ventricle
LVAD	left ventricular assisted device
LVOT	left ventricular outflow tract
MAPCA	major aorto-pulmonary collateral arteries
MI	myocardial infarction
MIP	maximum intensity projection
MPR	multiplanar reconstruction
MR	magnetic resonance
MRA	magnetic resonance angiography
NECT	nonenhanced computed tomography
OM	obtuse marginal
PA	pulmonary artery
PAPVR	partial anomalous pulmonary venous return
PCI	percutaneous coronary intervention
PDA	posterior descending artery; patent ductus arteriosus
PFO	patent foramen ovale
PLB	posterolateral branch
PV	pulmonary vein
RA	right atrium
RCA	right coronary artery
RBBB	right bundle branch block
RLL	right lower lobe
RML	right middle lobe
ROI	region of interest
RUL	right upper lobe
RV	right ventricle

RVOT	right ventricular outflow tract
SA	sinoatrial
SAM	systolic anterior motion
SANodal	sinoatrial nodal
SSFP	steady-state free perfusion
SVC	superior vena cava
T1WI	T1-weighted image
T2WI	T2-weighted image
T1+Gad	T1-weighted image plus gadolinium enhancement
TAPVR	total anomalous pulmonary venous return
TGA	transposition of great arteries
TOF	tetralogy of Fallot
US	ultrasound
VSD	ventricular septal defect
XA	x-ray angiography

Part 1   Normal Anatomy

History

▶ None

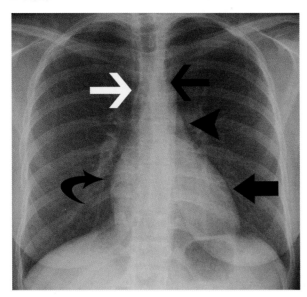

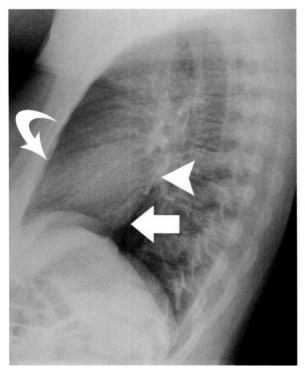

Case 1 Cardiac Anatomy

Findings

- ► Border-forming structures
  - ■ Frontal view:
    - ◆ Left upper border (black arrow): Left subclavian artery, aortic arch (aortic knob)
    - ◆ Left middle border (black arrowhead): Main pulmonary artery (pulmonary trunk), left arterial appendage
    - ◆ Left lower border (black block arrow): Left ventricle
    - ◆ Right upper border (white arrow): Innominate vein and superior vena cava or innominate artery and ascending aorta
    - ◆ Right lower border (black curved arrow): Right atrial appendage and right atrium, inferior vena cava
  - ■ Lateral view:
    - ◆ Anterior lower border (white curved arrow): Right ventricle
    - ◆ Posterior upper border (white arrowhead): Left atrium and pulmonary veins
    - ◆ Posterior lower border (white block arrow): Left ventricle (sometimes right atrium), inferior vena cava
- ► Cardiac position: Normally, approximately one-third of the heart lies to the right and two-thirds of the heart lies to the left of the midline
- ► Cardiac size
  - ■ Evaluated either subjectively (most common) or by measuring the cardiothoracic ratio
    - ◆ Cardiothoracic ratio = maximum transverse cardiac diameter to transverse thoracic diameter; should be ≤ 0.55
  - ■ Technical factors, such as rotation and projection, need to be taken into account
- ► Cardiac valves
  - ■ Mitral and aortic valves are in continuity
    - ◆ The aortic valve lies above the mitral valve
    - ◆ Best visualized by using an imaginary line drawn either in the frontal view (from the left atrial appendage to the point of intersection of the right atrium and diaphragm) or the lateral view (from the carina to the point of intersection of the sternum and left diaphragm)
  - ■ Tricuspid and pulmonary valves are separated significantly
    - ◆ Tricuspid valve is the most inferior valve

Further Readings

Gibbs JM et al. Lines and stripes: where did they go?—From conventional radiography to CT. *Radiographics*. 2007;27(1):33–48.

Lipton MJ et al. How to approach cardiac diagnosis from the chest radiograph. *Radiol Clin North Am.* 2004;42(3):487–495.

History

▸ None

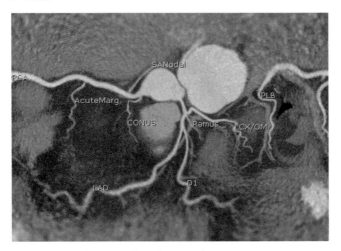

Figure 2-1 Two-dimensional coronary map

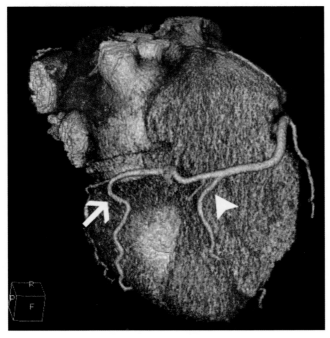

Figure 2-2 Multiplanar reconstruction of the inferior cardiac border

Case 2 Normal Coronary Arteries

Findings

- ▶ Right and left aortic coronary sinuses of Valsalva give rise to the right coronary artery (RCA) and left coronary artery (LCA)
- ▶ The RCA courses rightward and posterior to the right ventricular outflow tract (RVOT), in the right atrioventricular (AV) groove, and gives off multiple branches
  - ▪ Conus branch—first branch of the RCA (exists 50% of the time), which supplies the RVOT; otherwise, arises from a separate origin from the right coronary sinus
  - ▪ Sinoatrial nodal (SANodal) branch—second branch (60%), which supplies the sinoatrial node; otherwise, arises from the left circumflex (LCx) coronary artery
  - ▪ Anterior branches—supply the lateral wall of the right ventricle (RV)
  - ▪ Acute marginal (AcuteMarg) artery—arises from the mid- to the distal RCA; supplies the free wall of the RV
  - ▪ Posterolateral branch (PLB—arrow) and posterior descending artery (PDA—arrowhead)—last two branches of the RCA, which may supply the posterior interventricular septum; indicates right dominance (85%)
    - ◆ If left dominant (7.5%), the PLB and PDA arise from the LCx coronary artery
    - ◆ If codominant (7.5%), the PLB and PDA arise from the LCx coronary artery and RCA, respectively
    - ◆ AV nodal branch arises from the PDA and supplies the AV node
- ▶ LCA begins as the left main (LM) coronary artery, courses leftward and posterior to the RVOT, and bifurcates into the left anterior descending (LAD) and LCx coronary arteries or trifurcates into the LAD and LCx coronary arteries and the ramus intermedius
  - ▪ LAD coronary artery courses in the anterior interventricular groove and gives off diagonal and septal branches
    - ◆ Diagonal (D) branches—supply the anterior wall of the left ventricle (LV); branches are numbered from the LCx (e.g., D1 is the first diagonal branch after the LCx)
      - • Ramus intermedius—a variant, courses similarly to the first diagonal branch
    - ◆ Septal branches—supply the anterior interventricular septum; branches are numbered from the LCx
  - ▪ LCx coronary artery courses in the left AV groove and gives off obtuse marginal (OM) branches
    - ◆ OM branches—supply the lateral wall of the LV

Further Readings

Kini S et al. Normal and variant coronary arterial and venous anatomy on high-resolution CT angiography. *AJR Am J Roentgenol.* 2007;188(6):1665–1674.
Pannu HK et al. Current concepts in multi-detector row CT evaluation of the coronary arteries: principles, techniques, and anatomy. *Radiographics.* 2003;23 Spec No:S111–S125.

History

▶ None

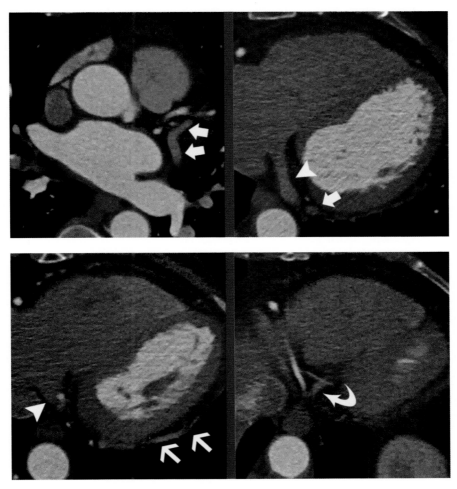

Case 3 Normal Coronary Veins

Findings

- ► Most accompany coronary arteries and their branches
- ► Most coronary veins drain into the coronary sinus, which drains into the right atrium (RA)
- ► Coronary sinus (arrowheads)
  - Wide vein that courses in the posterior AV groove
  - Accompanies the LCx coronary artery (which continues in the posterior AV groove if there is left coronary dominance)
  - Receives (proximally to distally) the greater cardiac vein (left coronary vein), oblique vein of the left atrium (LA) (oblique vein of Marshall), posterior vein of the LV (posterolateral vein), middle cardiac vein, and small cardiac vein (right coronary vein)
  - Great cardiac vein (block arrows)—arises from the apex, courses upward in the anterior interventricular groove accompanying the LAD coronary artery, and continues in the left AV groove
    - Tributaries from the LA, RV, and LV; the left marginal vein is one of the tributaries
  - Oblique vein of LA—courses obliquely posterior to the LA
  - Posterior vein of the LV (arrows)—courses along the lateral wall of the LV
  - Middle cardiac vein (curved arrow)—arises from the apex and courses upward in the inferior interventricular groove accompanying the PDA
  - Small cardiac vein—arises from the RA and RV, courses along the right margin of the heart accompanying the acute marginal artery, and continues in the right AV groove
- ► Other coronary veins drain directly into the RA
  - Anterior cardiac veins (anterior veins of the RV)—three or four small vessels arise in front of the RV

Further Readings

Kini S et al. Normal and variant coronary arterial and venous anatomy on high-resolution CT angiography. *AJR Am J Roentgenol.* 2007;188(6):1665–1674.

Singh JP et al. The coronary venous anatomy: a segmental approach to aid cardiac resynchronization therapy. *J Am Coll Cardiol.* 2005;46(1):68–74.

Case 4

History

▶ None

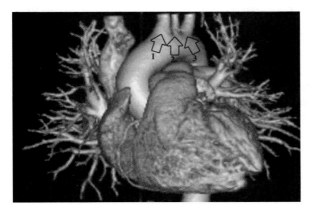

Figure 4-1 Anterior three-dimensional volumetric reconstruction

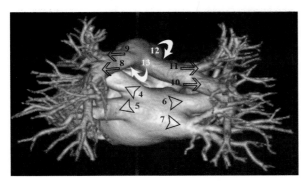

Figure 4-2 Posterior three-dimensional volumetric reconstruction

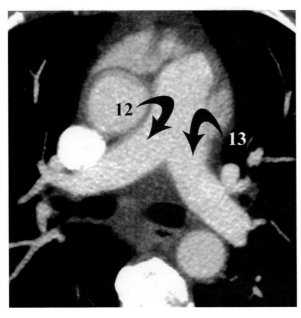

9

Case 4 Great Vessels

Findings

- Aorta: three segments—ascending, transverse (or arch), and descending
  - Ascending segment
    - Arises from the LV and extends to the origin of the innominate artery
    - Aortic root—proximal portion of the aorta—includes the aortic valve, annulus, and sinuses of Valsalva
  - Transverse segment or aortic arch
    - Begins at the origin of the innominate artery, courses from right to left, anterior to posterior in the superior mediastinum, and ends at the ligamentum or ductus arteriosum
    - Gives off the innominate or brachiocephalic artery (block arrow 1), left common carotid artery (CCA) (block arrow 2), and left subclavian artery (SCA) (block arrow 3)
      - Aortic isthmus—distal aortic arch after the origin of the left SCA
  - Descending aorta
    - Begins at the ligamentum or ductus arteriosum
    - Gives off the intercostal arteries and bronchial arteries
- Pulmonary arteries (PAs): Branches usually follow corresponding bronchial courses
  - Main PA arises from the RVOT, anterior and to the left of the ascending aorta, and bifurcates into the right and left PAs; the right PA is longer and larger than the left
    - Right PA (curved arrow 12) courses horizontally and posteriorly to the ascending aorta, superior vena cava, and right superior pulmonary vein (PV), and anteriorly to the right upper lobe (RUL) bronchus, and bifurcates into two branches
      - Truncus anterior or right ascending PA (arrow 11)—supplies the RUL
      - Interlobar or descending PA (arrow 10)—supplies the right middle lobe (RML) and right lower lobe (RLL)
    - Left PA (curved arrow 13) courses higher than the right PA, superiorly to the left main bronchus, and bifurcates into two branches
      - Left ascending PA (arrow 9)—supplies the left upper lobe (LUL)
      - Interlobar or descending PA (arrow 8)—supplies the lingula and left lower lobe (LLL)
- Pulmonary veins (PVs)
  - Four main PVs with four ostia inserting obliquely into the LA are most often seen (70%)
    - Right superior PV (arrowhead 7)—drains RUL and RML PVs
    - Right inferior PV (arrowhead 6)—drains RLL PV
    - Left superior PV (arrowhead 4)—drains LUL and lingular PVs
    - Left inferior PV (arrowhead 5)—drains LLL PV
  - Other anatomical variations:
    - Common ostium (from two PVs) inserting into the LA
      - More common on the left
    - Additional PV(s) inserting into the LA
      - More common on the right
      - Additional PV from the RML is associated with the occurrence of atrial fibrillation

Further Readings

Cronin P et al. MDCT of the left atrium and pulmonary veins in planning radiofrequency ablation for atrial fibrillation: a how-to guide. *AJR Am J Roentgenol.* 2004;183(3):767–778.

Goo HW et al. CT of congenital heart disease: normal anatomy and typical pathologic conditions. *Radiographics.* 2003;23 Spec No:S147–S165.

History

▸ None

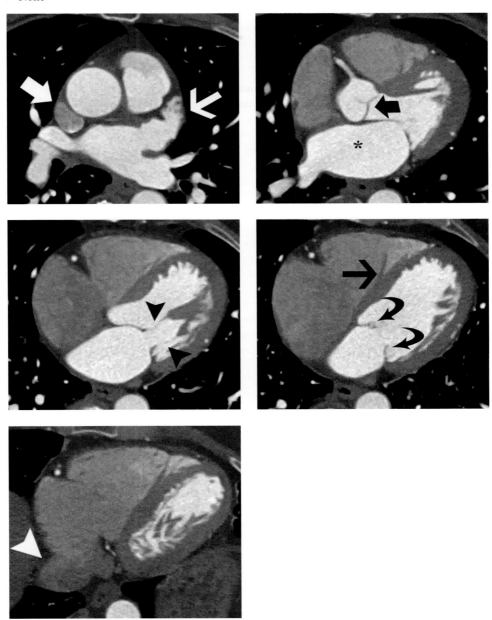

Case 5   Cardiac Chambers and Valves

Findings

▶ Four cardiac chambers
- Right atrium (RA)
  - Receives deoxygenated blood from the systemic circulation via the superior vena cava (SVC) (white block arrow), inferior vena cava (IVC) (white arrowhead), and coronary sinus; the blood exits the tricuspid valve
  - Crista terminalis—vertical ridge extending from the SVC to the IVC—allows differentiation between the RA and LA
  - Interatrial septum—includes the fossa ovalis (closed foramen ovale); separates the RA from the LA
- Left atrium (LA) (asterisk)
  - Receives oxygenated blood from the pulmonary circulation via PVs; the blood exits the mitral valve
  - Most superior and posterior cardiac chamber
  - Left atrial appendage (white arrow)—trabeculated cavity anterior and superior to the LV
- Right ventricle (RV)
  - Receives deoxygenated blood from the RA via the tricuspid valve; blood exits to the main PA via pulmonary valve
  - Most anterior cardiac chamber with heavy trabeculation
  - Three papillary muscles—anterior, posterior, septal
  - Interventricular septum—separates the RV from the LV
  - Moderator band (black arrow)—attaches the anterior papillary muscle to the interventricular septum near the RV apex; contains the right bundle branch
- Left ventricle (LV)
  - Receives oxygenated blood from the LA via the mitral valve; blood exits to the aorta via the aortic valve
  - Thicker myocardium than the RV, with less trabeculation
  - Two papillary muscles—anterior, posterior
▶ Four cardiac valves—regulate unidirectional blood flow through the four cardiac chambers
- Two semilunar valves
  - Pulmonary valve
    - Separates the RV from the main PA
    - Three cusps (left, right, anterior)
  - Aortic valve (block black arrow)
    - Separates the LV from the aorta
    - Three cusps (right, left, posterior)
    - RCA takes off from the right sinus
    - LCA takes off from the left sinus
    - Posterior sinus is a noncoronary sinus
- Two AV valves
  - Tricuspid valve
    - Separates the RA from the RV
    - Three leaflets (anterior, posterior, septal) attached to the annulus fibrosus dexter cordis
  - Mitral valve (curved arrows)
    - Separates the LA from the LV
    - Two leaflets (anterior, posterior) attached to the annulus fibrosus sinister cordis
  - Each leaflet is connected to ventricular papillary muscles by chordae tendinae (black arrowheads)
  - Each leaflet is continuous with the other leaflet(s) at the bases by commissures

Further Readings

Broderick LS et al. Anatomic pitfalls of the heart and pericardium. *Radiographics.* 2005;25(2):441–453.
O'Brien JP et al. Anatomy of the heart at multidetector CT: what the radiologist needs to know. *Radiographics.* 2007;27(6):1569–1582.

Part 2

**Congenital Heart Disease—
Coronary and Great Vessels**

History

▸ None

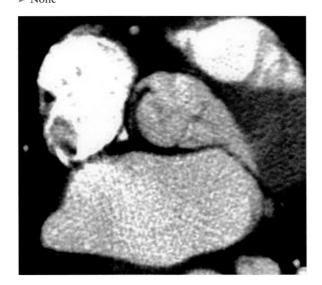

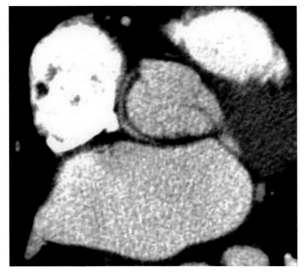

Case 6 Benign Anomalous Left Circumflex Coronary Artery

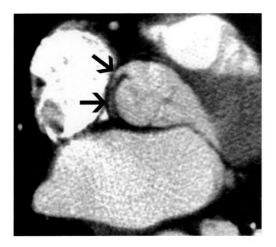

Findings

- LCx coronary artery arises from a separate ostium within the right sinus of Valsalva or as a proximal branch of the RCA, courses posteriorly (arrow) and leftward between the atria and noncoronary cusp of the aortic valve, and traverses the left AV groove
- The LAD artery originates directly from the left sinus of Valsalva without a "true" LM segment of the LCA

Differential Diagnosis

- Benign anomalous origin of the RCA
- Coronary artery fistula
- Sinoatrial (SA) node branch

Teaching Points

- The groove between the atria and the noncoronary cusp of the aortic valve is normally vessel-free; therefore, if a vessel is identified, an anomalous LCx coronary artery or a benign variant of an anomalous origin of the RCA must be considered
  - A benign variant of an anomalous origin of the RCA originates from the left sinus of Valsalva and courses posteriorly and toward the right
- Coronary artery fistula and the SA node branch have a normal LCx coronary artery as a branch of the LCA

Management

- None; usually a benign finding noted incidentally on cardiac computed tomographic angiography (CTA)

Further Readings

Dodd JD et al. Congenital anomalies of coronary artery origin in adults: 64-MDCT appearance. *AJR Am J Roentgenol.* 2007;188(2):W138–W146.

Kim SY et al. Coronary artery anomalies: classification and ECG-gated multi-detector row CT findings with angiographic correlation. *Radiographics.* 2006;26(2):317–333.

History

▸ None

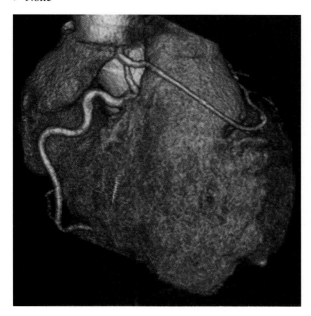

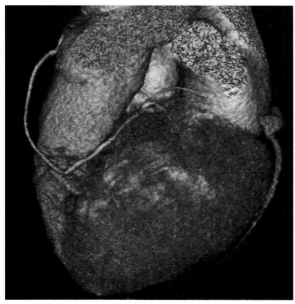

Case 7 Benign Anomalous Left Coronary Artery

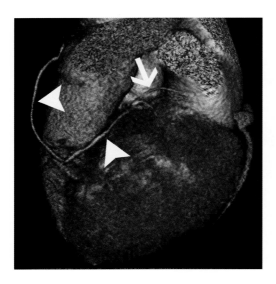

Findings

- LM segment of the LCA arises from the right sinus of Valsalva or from the RCA, courses anteriorly to the RVOT (arrowheads), and becomes the origin of the LAD (*minute and not seen in the above image*) and LCx (arrow) coronary arteries
- Left sinus of Valsalva lacks a coronary ostium

Differential Diagnosis

- Malignant, anomalous LCA
- Anomalous origin of the LAD artery
- Anomalous LCx artery
- Coronary artery fistula

Teaching Points

- Malignant variant of an anomalous LCA courses between the PA and the aorta
- Both anomalous origin of the LAD and anomalous LCx arteries have an absent LM segment of the LCA but an intact coronary ostium in the left sinus of Valsalva
- In a coronary artery fistula, the involved coronary artery is dilated and tortuous and may mimic an anomalous LCA; there is an intact coronary ostium in the left sinus of Valsalva

Management

- None; usually a benign congenital finding noted incidentally on catheter angiography or cardiac CTA (1%–2% of the general population)

Further Readings

Dodd JD et al. Congenital anomalies of coronary artery origin in adults: 64-MDCT appearance. *AJR Am J Roentgenol.* 2007;188(2):W138–W146.

Kim SY et al. Coronary artery anomalies: classification and ECG-gated multi-detector row CT findings with angiographic correlation. *Radiographics.* 2006;26(2):317–333.

History

▶ Two 18-year-old men who presented with chest pain during exercise.

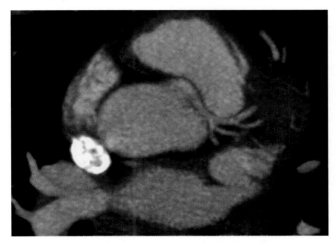

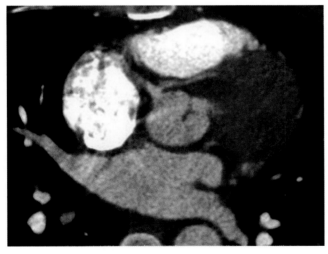

Case 8 Malignant Anomalous Left Coronary Artery

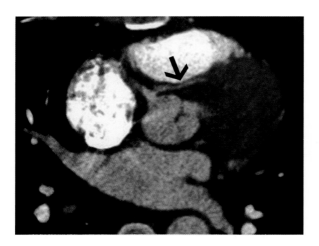

Findings

- LM segment of the LCA arises from the right sinus of Valsalva or from the RCA (arrow), courses between the PA and the aortic root (interarterial), and becomes the origin of the LAD and LCx arteries
- Left sinus of Valsalva lacks a coronary ostium

Differential Diagnosis

- Benign anomalous LCA
- Other coronary anomalies (e.g., anomalous origin of the RCA, LAD, or LCx artery)
- Coronary artery fistula

Teaching Points

- Benign variant of anomalous LCA courses anteriorly to the RVOT
- Other coronary anomalies usually have an intact coronary ostium in the left sinus of Valsalva compared to anomalous LCA
- Epidemiology: Children and young adults
- Presentation: Myocardial ischemia, heart failure, ventricular arrhythmia, or sudden death, usually during or after exercise
  - Due to the acute angle of the ostium, stretch of the intramural segment, and compression between the commissure of the right and left coronary cusps

Management

- Coronary artery bypass graft (CABG) surgery or reimplantation of the anomalous coronary artery to the appropriate coronary sinus

Further Readings

Dodd JD et al. Congenital anomalies of coronary artery origin in adults: 64-MDCT appearance. *AJR Am J Roentgenol.* 2007;188(2):W138–W146.

Kim SY et al. Coronary artery anomalies: classification and ECG-gated multi-detector row CT findings with angiographic correlation. *Radiographics.* 2006;26(2):317–333.

History

► None

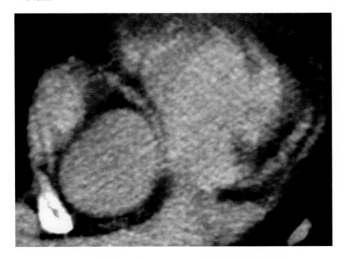

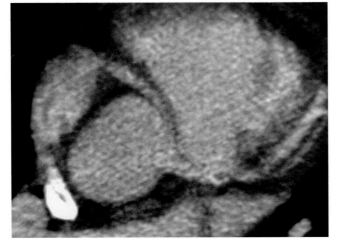

Case 9 Malignant Anomalous Origin of Right Coronary Artery

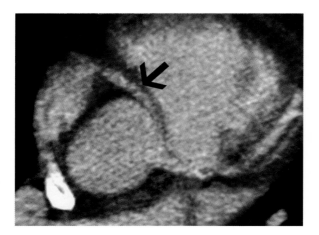

Findings
- ► RCA arises from the left sinus of Valsalva or LM segment of the LCA, courses between the PA and aortic root (interarterial) (arrow), and traverses distally in the right AV groove
- ► Right sinus of Valsalva lacks a coronary ostium

Differential Diagnosis
- ► Anomalous origin of the RCA, benign
- ► Other coronary anomalies (e.g., anomalous origin of the LCA, LAD, or LCx artery)
- ► Coronary artery fistula

Teaching Points
- ► Benign variant (less common than the malignant variant) of the RCA anomaly arises from the left sinus of Valsalva or the LM segment of the LCA and courses posteriorly to the aortic root
- ► Other coronary anomalies usually have an intact coronary ostium in the right sinus of Valsalva
- ► Epidemiology: Young adults
- ► Presentation: Arrhythmia or sudden death during/after exercise
  - ■ Malignant coronary anomalies (include the malignant variant of anomalous LCA) are the second most common cause of young adult death

Management
- ► Controversial; medical management with a ß-blocker or surgical revascularization

Further Readings

Dodd JD et al. Congenital anomalies of coronary artery origin in adults: 64-MDCT appearance. *AJR Am J Roentgenol.* 2007;188(2):W138–W146.

Kim SY et al. Coronary artery anomalies: classification and ECG-gated multi-detector row CT findings with angiographic correlation. *Radiographics.* 2006;26(2):317–333.

History

► None

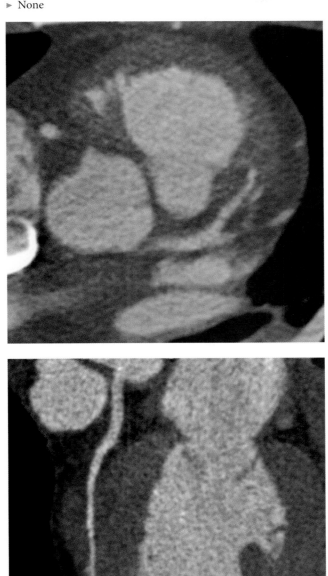

Case 10 Myocardial Bridging

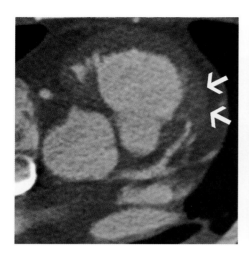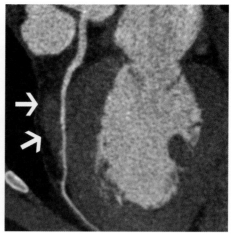

Findings

▶ A band of myocardial muscle (arrows) overlying a segment of coronary artery
▶ A segment of the coronary artery courses intramyocardially and resurfaces to the epicardial fat
▶ Most common in the middle segment of the LAD artery (as in this case), followed by LCx and RCA
▶ Electrocardiography (ECG)-gated reconstruction can be performed during the systolic and diastolic phases to assess maximal luminal narrowing and dilation, respectively

Differential Diagnosis

▶ Coronary artery disease
▶ Cardiac tumor
▶ Hypertrophic cardiomyopathy

Teaching Points

▶ Segment of the coronary artery proximal to the myocardial bridge is predisposed to atherosclerotic changes, while the tunneled area is relatively protected
▶ Cardiac tumor may invade epicardial fat and engulf the coronary arteries
▶ Hypertrophic cardiomyopathy may mimic myocardial bridging due to asymmetrical enlargement of the myocardium partially engulfing the coronary artery
▶ Presentation: Most cases are asymptomatic; symptoms include angina, myocardial infarction, life-threatening arrhythmias, and even sudden death
  ▪ Due to marked systolic compression of an epicardial coronary arterial segment by the overlying myocardium

Management

▶ None; usually asymptomatic
▶ Medical (ß-blocker or calcium channel blocker) or surgical (coronary revascularization or septal myomectomy) treatment in symptomatic patients

Further Reading

Konen E et al. Myocardial bridging, a common anatomical variant rather than a congenital anomaly. *Semin Ultrasound CT MR*. 2008;29(3):195–203.

History

▶ A 1-month-old infant with clinical symptoms of congestive heart failure

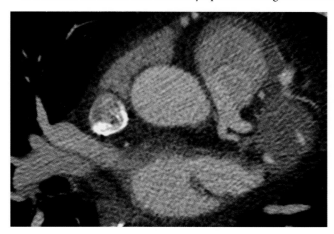

Figure 11-1   Image courtesy of Jacob Kirsch,
MD (Cleveland Clinics, Ft. Lauderdale, Florida)

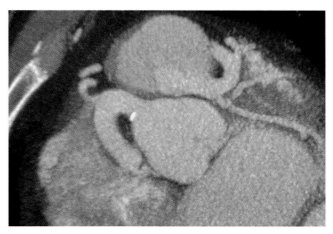

Figure 11-2   Image courtesy of Jacob Kirsch,
MD (Cleveland Clinics, Ft. Lauderdale, Florida)

Case 11 Bland-White-Garland Syndrome

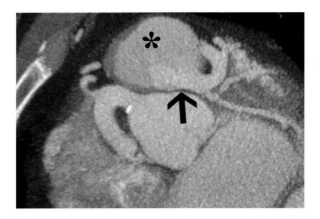

Findings

▶ An anomalous coronary artery, usually the LM segment of the LCA (arrow), arises from the PA (asterisk) and courses normally in the anterior interventricular groove

Differential Diagnosis

▶ Other coronary artery anomalies
▶ Coronary artery fistula

Teaching Points

▶ Also known as *anomalous left coronary artery from the pulmonary artery* (ALCAPA)
▶ Other coronary artery anomalies do not arise from the PA
▶ In coronary artery fistula, the LCA arises from the coronary ostium correctly, although abnormal branch vessels of the fistula may connect to the PA
▶ Most patients usually present as infants with heart failure; in rare cases, adults may present with angina, myocardial infarction, or heart failure
▶ Lower PA pressure results in the coronary steal phenomenon, which in turn results in ischemia

Management

▶ In infants, reimplantation or intrapulmonary conduit of the anomalous coronary artery to the aorta can be performed
▶ In adults, the anomalous LCA can be ligated and CABG can be performed

Further Readings

Cowles RA et al. Bland-White-Garland syndrome of anomalous left coronary artery arising from the pulmonary artery (ALCAPA): a historical review. *Pediatr Radiol.* 2007;37(9):890–895.
Kim SY et al. Coronary artery anomalies: classification and ECG-gated multi-detector row CT findings with angiographic correlation. *Radiographics.* 2006;26(2):317–333.

History

▶ None

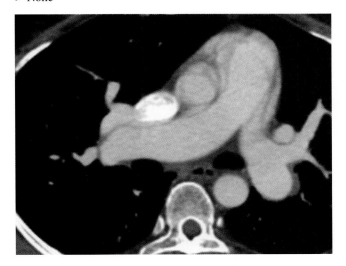

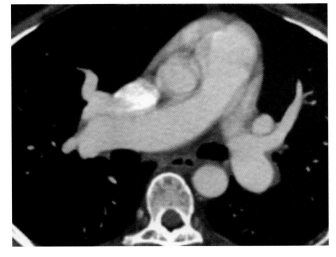

Case 12 Partial Anomalous Pulmonary Venous Return

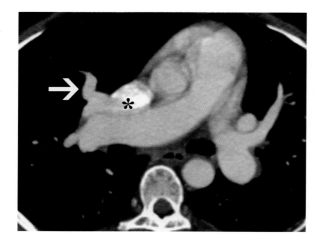

Findings

- One or more, but not all, of the PVs (arrow) drain into a systemic vein instead of the LA, resulting in a left-to-right shunt
- Right lung most frequently drains into the SVC (asterisk)
- Left lung most frequently drains into the left brachiocephalic vein
- Other systemic veins into which anomalous PVs may drain include IVC, hepatic veins, portal veins, azygos vein, coronary sinus, and RA

Differential Diagnosis

- Left SVC
- Pulmonary varix
- Left superior intercostal vein

Teaching Points

- Isolated partial anomalous pulmonary venous return (PAPVR) of the right upper lobe draining to the SVC is the most frequent type of PAPVR and is associated with the sinus venosus type of atrial septal defect (ASD)
- Left-to-right shunt is usually hemodynamically inconsequential and asymptomatic unless associated with congestive heart disease (CHD) or scimitar (venolobar) syndrome

Management

- None; usually an incidental finding on cross-sectional imaging
- Consider surgical or percutaneous closure in patients with ASD

Further Readings

Demos TC et al. Venous anomalies of the thorax. *AJR Am J Roentgenol.* 2004;182(5):1139–1150.
Haramati LB et al. Computed tomography of partial anomalous pulmonary venous connection in adults. *J Comput Assist Tomogr.* 2003;27(5):743–749.
Konen E et al. Congenital pulmonary venolobar syndrome: spectrum of helical CT findings with emphasis on computerized reformatting. *Radiographics.* 2003;23(5):1175–1184.

History

▸ None

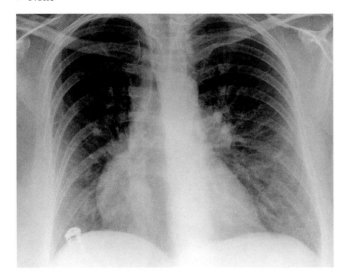

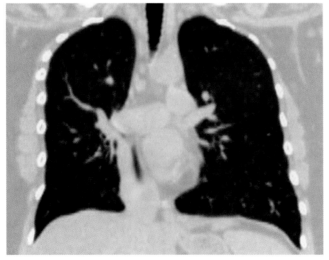

Case 13 Scimitar Syndrome

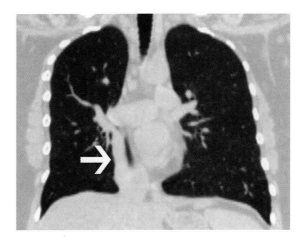

Findings

▶ Curved anomalous pulmonary vein (arrow) draining into the IVC and traversing the right medial cardiophrenic sulcus; resembles a Turkish sword (hence the term *scimitar sign*)
▶ Other findings include right lung hypoplasia, rightward shift of the mediastinum, prominent right atrium, pulmonary vascular congestion, and an abnormal systemic arterial supply to the right lung base

Differential Diagnosis

▶ Other types of PAPVR
▶ Meandering pulmonary vein
▶ Pulmonary sequestration
▶ Swyer-James syndrome (hypoplastic lung)

Teaching Points

▶ Scimitar syndrome is a type of right-sided PAPVR (*see Case12: Partial Anomalous Pulmonary Venous Return*)
▶ Also known as *hypogenic lung syndrome* or *venolobar syndrome*
▶ Associated with cardiac anomalies (25%); ASD is most common
▶ Symptoms dependent on age of presentation and size of the left-to-right shunt
  ▪ Neonates: right-sided heart failure, pulmonary hypertension
  ▪ Children: recurrent infections
  ▪ Adults: usually asymptomatic

Management

▶ If the patient is symptomatic, surgical resection can be performed
▶ Consider presurgical embolization of the systemic arterial supply
▶ Cardiac surgery or intervention for associated cardiac anomalies

Further Reading

Berrocal T et al. Congenital anomalies of the tracheobronchial tree, lung, and mediastinum: embryology, radiology, and pathology. *Radiographics*. 2004;24(1):e17.

History

▶ None

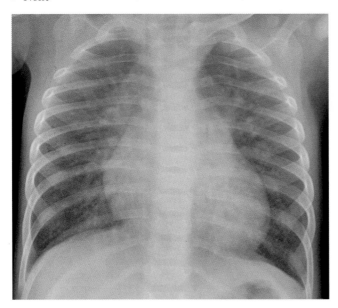

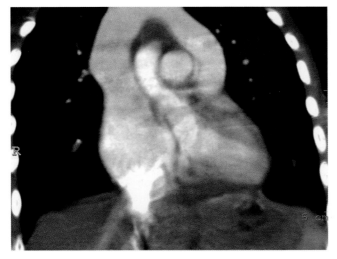

Case 14 Total Anomalous Pulmonary Venous Return

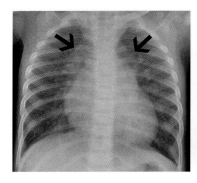 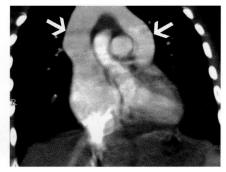

Findings

- ▶ Supracardiac (type 1): Common PV drains superiorly via the vertical vein into the left innominate vein
  - ▪ Chest x-ray (CXR): Frontal view: "Snowman" heart (arrows), cardiomegaly, shunt vascularity
- ▶ Cardiac (type 2): Common PV drains into the coronary sinus or RA
  - ▪ CXR: Frontal view: Cardiomegaly, shunt vascularity
- ▶ Infracardiac (type 3): Common PV drains into the portal vein, ductus venosus, or IVC below the diaphragm
  - ▪ CXR: Frontal view: Normal heart size, pulmonary edema (venous obstruction by diaphragmatic hiatus)
- ▶ Mixed (type 4): Mixture of types 1 to 3

Differential Diagnosis

- ▶ Partial anomalous pulmonary venous return—multiple vessels
- ▶ Cor triatriatum
- ▶ Hypoplastic left heart syndrome

Teaching Points

- ▶ Extracardiac left-to-right shunt
- ▶ All types are associated with either PDA or ASD, allowing an obligatory right-to-left shunt for viability
- ▶ Epidemiology: Neonates
- ▶ Presentation: Progressive congestive heart failure (type 1 and 2) or severe cyanosis at birth (type 3)

Management

- ▶ Medical treatment with prostaglandin E1 or extracorporeal membrane oxygenation (ECMO) to improve oxygenation
- ▶ Surgical anastomosis of the PV to the LA and ligation of other abnormal pulmonary venous veins are required for viability

Further Readings

Ferguson EC et al. Classic imaging signs of congenital cardiovascular abnormalities. *Radiographics.* 2007;27(5):1323–1334.

Zylak CJ et al. Developmental lung anomalies in the adult: radiologic–pathologic correlation. *Radiographics.* 2002;22 Spec No:S25–S43.

History

▶ A 69-year-old male with worsening shortness of breath

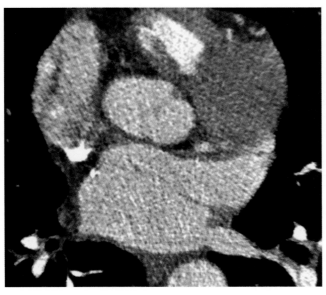

Figure 15-1   Image courtesy of Jeffrey S. Mueller, MD (Allegheny General Hospital, Pittsburgh, Pennsylvania)

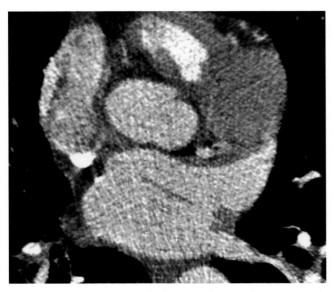

Figure 15-2   Image courtesy of Jeffrey S. Mueller, MD (Allegheny General Hospital, Pittsburgh, Pennsylvania)

Case 15 Cor Triatriatum

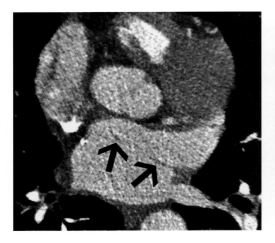 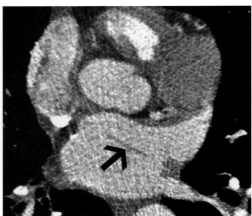

Findings

- ► A membrane (arrows) separating the left atrium into anterior and posterior compartments
    - ▪ Pulmonary veins drain into the posterior compartment
    - ▪ Left atrial appendage and mitral valve arise from the anterior compartment
- ► Depending on the size of the defect within the membrane is small, pulmonary venous hypertension may result

Differential Diagnosis

- ► Submitral ring or web
- ► Anomalous pulmonary venous return, total
- ► Cor triatriatum dextra

Teaching Points

- ► Also known as *cor triatriatum sinister*
- ► Membrane best visualized on conventional echocardiography
- ► Severity of symptoms depends on the size of the defect within the membrane
- ► Symptoms resemble those of mitral valve stenosis

Management

- ► If the patient is symptomatic, surgical resection of the membrane can be performed

Further Readings

Saremi F et al. Multidetector computed tomography (MDCT) in diagnosis of "cor triatriatum sinister."
J Cardiovasc Comput Tomogr. 2007;1(3):172–174.
Su CS et al. Usefulness of multidetector-row computed tomography in evaluating adult cor triatriatum.
Tex Heart Inst J. 2008;35(3):349–351.

History

▶ None

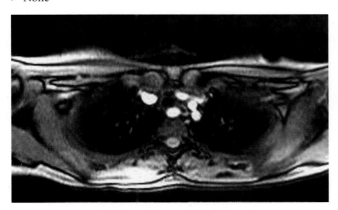

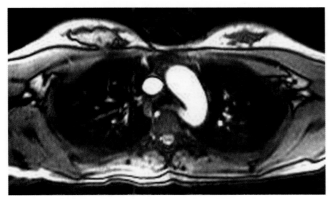

Case 16 Aberrant Right Subclavian Artery

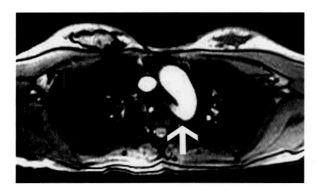

Findings

▶ Computed tomography/magnetic resonance (CT/MR): Last arterial branch (arrow) arises from a four-branch aortic arch, courses between the esophagus and the vertebral spine, and becomes the right subclavian artery
  - The arterial origin is often dilated, a condition called the *diverticulum of Kommerell*
▶ Esophagram: Lateral view: Posterior indentation of the esophagus

Differential Diagnosis

▶ Mediastinal masses (e.g., lymph node, neurogenic tumor, substernal thyroid)
▶ Other aortic anomalies (e.g., double aortic arch, right aortic arch)
▶ Aortic aneurysm

Teaching Points

▶ Most common substantial congenital anomaly of the aortic arch
▶ Does not form a vascular ring
▶ Presentation: Asymptomatic; rarely, compression of the posterior esophagus may result in dysphagia lusoria

Management

▶ None; usually a benign congenital finding (0.5% of the general population)

Further Readings

Franquet T et al. The retrotracheal space: normal anatomic and pathologic appearances. *Radiographics*. 2002;22 Spec No:S231–S246.
Raider L et al. The retrotracheal triangle. *Radiographics*. 1990;10(6):1055–1079.

History

▶ None

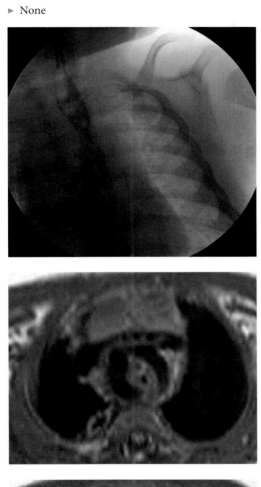

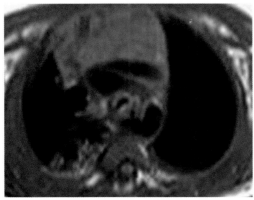

Case 17 Double Aortic Arch

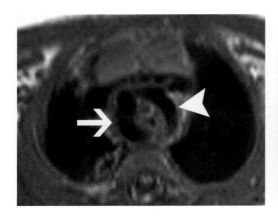 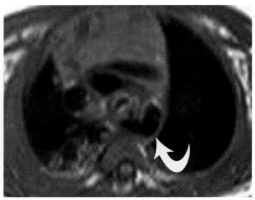

Findings

- ▶ Esophagram:
  - ▪ Frontal view: Bilateral indentations of the esophagus, usually near the superior right arch and inferior left arch
  - ▪ Lateral view: Posterior esophagus indentation at the level of the aortic arch
- ▶ CT/MR:
  - ▪ Left (arrowhead) and right (arrow) aortic arches arise from the ascending aorta and join to form a single descending aorta (curved arrow)
  - ▪ Respective carotid and subclavian arteries arise from each aortic arch
  - ▪ Complete vascular ring encircles both the trachea and the esophagus
    - ◆ Either the right (75%) or left (20%) aortic arch may appear dominant; the smaller arch may be atretic
    - ◆ Symmetric aortic arch (5%)

Differential Diagnosis

- ▶ Other arch anomalies (e.g., right aortic arch with aberrant left subclavian artery)
- ▶ Left pulmonary artery sling
- ▶ Innominate artery compression syndrome
- ▶ Mediastinal mass

Teaching Points

- ▶ Persistence of congenital left and right fourth aortic arches
- ▶ The most common types of vascular ring are the double aortic arch and the right aortic arch with left ligamentum arteriosum (85%–95% of cases)
- ▶ Associated with severe tracheobronchial anomalies (e.g., tracheomalacia, stenosis, webs, complete tracheal cartilage rings)
- ▶ Most common symptomatic vascular ring; symptoms include inspiratory stridor that worsens during feeding, usually developing during infancy

Management

- ▶ Thoracotomy can be performed through the opposite side of the dominant arch to ligate the nondominant arch and relieve the tracheal and esophageal compression

Further Reading

Lowe GM et al. Vascular rings: 10-year review of imaging. *Radiographics.* 1991;11(4):637–646.

History

▶ None

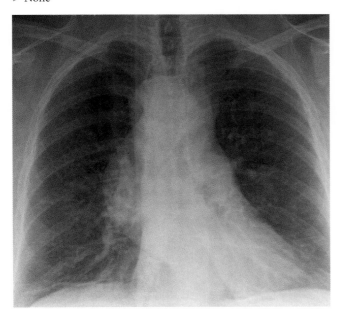

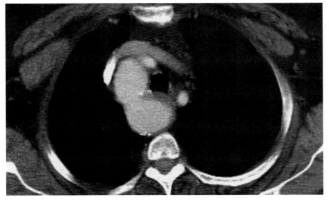

Case 18   Right Aortic Arch

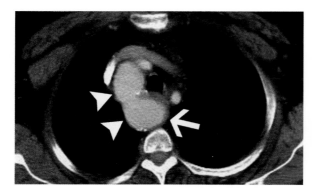

Findings

▶ CXR: Frontal view: Right paratracheal density with right-sided indentation of the trachea and tracheal deviation to the left
▶ Esophagram: Lateral view: Posterior indentation of the esophagus (in patients with aberrant left subclavian artery only)
▶ CT/MR: Most common types of branching patterns
   ▪ Right aortic arch with mirror image branching
   ▪ Right aortic arch (arrowheads) with aberrant left subclavian artery from the aortic arch (arrow)

Differential Diagnosis

▶ Other arch anomalies (e.g., double aortic arch)
▶ Aberrant right subclavian artery
▶ Mediastinal mass

Teaching Points

▶ Right aortic arch with an aberrant left subclavian artery is usually asymptomatic
   ▪ Symptoms (12%–25% of patients) are usually due to tight left ductus arteriosus (i.e., stridor) or a large diverticulum of Komerell (i.e., dysphagia)
▶ Right aortic arch with mirror image branching is associated with CHD (98%) (90% is tetralogy of Fallot [TOF])

Management

▶ None; usually an incidental finding
▶ If the patient is symptomatic, left thoracotomy to divide the ductus arteriosus can be performed

Further Reading

Franquet T et al. The retrotracheal space: normal anatomic and pathologic appearances. *Radiographics*. 2002;22 Spec No:S231–S246.

History

▶ None

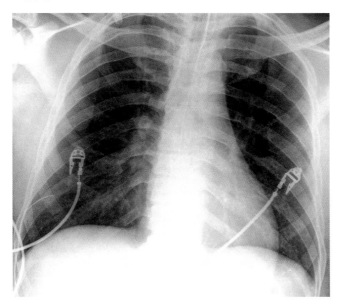

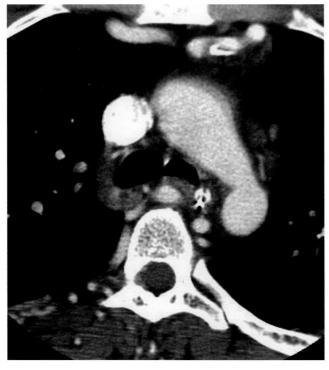

Case 19 Coarctation of Aorta

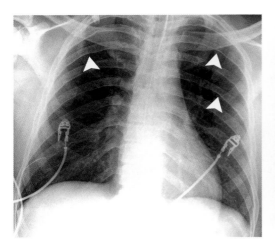 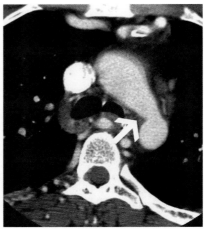

Findings

▶ CXR: Frontal view: Flow-limiting stenosis of the aorta resulting in poststenotic dilatation ("figure of 3" sign), rib notching (arrowheads), and LV hypertrophy
▶ Esophagram: Lateral view: reverse figure of 3 sign
▶ CT/MR:
  ▪ Focal narrowing (arrow) of the aorta (best visualized in an oblique three-dimensional volumetric-reconstruction view) with poststenotic dilatation of the descending aorta and collateral vessels
  ▪ Phase-contrast MR: Allows estimation of flow velocities, flow gradient, and collateral flow

Differential Diagnosis

▶ Pseudocoarctation
▶ Interrupted aortic arch
▶ Takayasu arteritis, chronic

Teaching Points

▶ Two types:
  ▪ Preductal or infantile-type (also known as *tubular hypoplasia*)
    ◆ Second most common cause of heart failure in infants
  ▪ Postductal or adult-type (also known as *localized coarctation*)
    ◆ Presentation: hypertension (HTN), diminished femoral pulses, and/or differential blood pressure between upper and lower extremities
▶ Associated with Turner's syndrome, Shone syndrome, ventricular septal defect (VSD), bicuspid aortic valve, and aneurysms of the circle of Willis

Management

▶ If the patient is symptomatic, surgical reconstruction or balloon angioplasty can be performed

Further Reading

Ferguson EC et al. Classic imaging signs of congenital cardiovascular abnormalities. *Radiographics*. 2007;27(5):1323–1334.

History

▶ A 31-year-old presents for follow-up imaging of a giant cell tumor

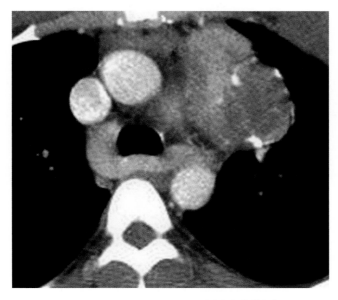

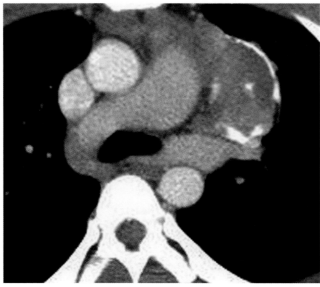

Case 20 Pulmonary Sling

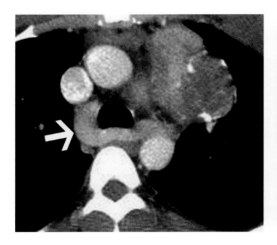 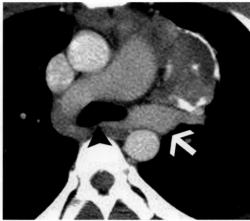

Findings

- ▶ CXR: Frontal view: Decreased left lung inflation and aeration
- ▶ Esophagram: Lateral view: Anterior indentation of the esophagus and posterior indentation of the trachea at the level of the carina
- ▶ CT/MR:
  - ▪ Left PA arises from the proximal right PA (arrows), courses leftward between the trachea and esophagus (arrowhead), and extend to the left hilum, posterior to the left mainstem bronchus
  - ▪ Left PA appears like a "sling" around the distal trachea and proximal right mainstem bronchus, displacing the trachea to the left

Differential Diagnosis

- ▶ Mediastinal mass, middle (e.g., bronchogenic cyst)
- ▶ Bronchial malformation (e.g., congenital lobar emphysema)
- ▶ Midline descending aorta-airway compression syndrome

Teaching Points

- ▶ Also known as *aberrant or anomalous origin of the left pulmonary artery*
- ▶ Pulmonary sling is the only vascular ring that leads to anterior indentation of the esophagus
- ▶ Associated with tracheal abnormalities (e.g., tracheomalacia, complete tracheal rings), abnormal pulmonary lobulation, and congenital heart disease
- ▶ Epidemiology: Usually neonates
- ▶ Presentation: Usually with severe stridor and hypoxia

Management

- ▶ If the patient is symptomatic, surgical reimplantation of the aberrant left PA to the main PA can be performed

Further Reading

Castañer E et al. Congenital and acquired pulmonary artery anomalies in the adult: radiologic overview. *Radiographics*. 2006;26(2):349–371.

Part 3   Great Vessel Disease

History

▶ A 40-year-old male present with acute chest pain

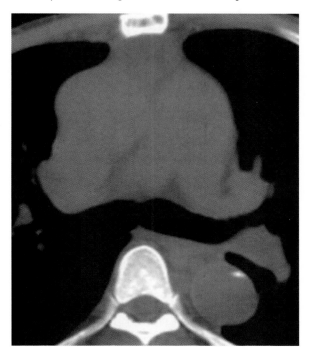

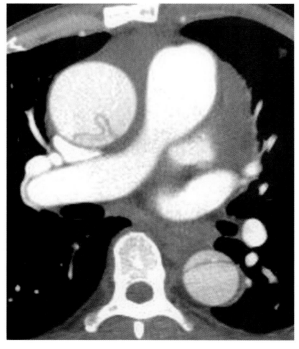

Case 21 Aortic Dissection

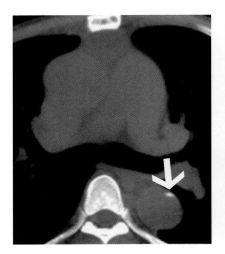 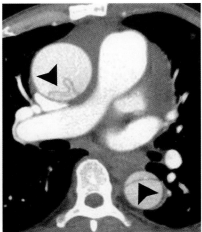

Findings

- ▶ CXR: Frontal view: Nonspecific; classically displaced intimal calcification
- ▶ CT:
  - ▪ Nonenhanced computed tomography (NECT): Aortic wall irregularity, calcification along the intimal flap (arrow), intramural or periaortic cresent of high attenuation (thrombosis)
  - ▪ Computed tomographic angiography (CTA): Intimal flap (arrowheads), entry site, compression of the true lumen by the false lumen, variable contrast attenuation in the false lumen (slow flow/thrombosis)
- ▶ MR: Intimal flap, variable signal intensity within the false lumen (depending on flow rate, thrombosis, and type of MR sequence)

Differential Diagnosis

- ▶ Thrombosed aortic aneurysm
- ▶ Intramural hematoma
- ▶ Penetrating atherosclerotic ulcer

Teaching Points

- ▶ A longitudinal partition of the aortic media, creating a true lumen (usually smaller and lined by intima) and a false lumen (lined by media)
- ▶ Two types (Stanford classification):
  - ▪ Type A: Ascending aorta ± descending aorta
  - ▪ Type B: Descending aorta only
- ▶ Etiology: Hypertension (70%), atherosclerosis, congenital (aortic coarctation, bicuspid valve, Marfan syndrome, Ehlers-Danlos syndrome), pregnancy
- ▶ Epidemiology:
  - ▪ Males (3:1) > females; 40–70 year old; most often African Americans
  - ▪ 21% mortality preadmission, 33% within 24 hours, 50% at 48 hours if untreated
- ▶ Presentation: Sudden onset of chest, neck/jaw, or back pain
- ▶ Complications: Pericardial dissection/cardiac tamponade, coronary/supra-aortic artery occlusion, aortic aneurysm/rupture, aortic valve damage, vascular ischemia

Management

- ▶ Type A: Surgical repair usually performed
- ▶ Type B: Medical therapy versus aortic stenting

Further Reading

Sebastià C et al. Aortic dissection: diagnosis and follow-up with helical CT. *Radiographics.* 1999;19(1):45–60.

History

▶ A 60-year-male presents with acute chest pain

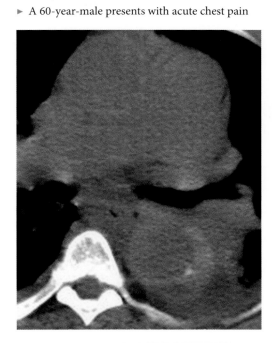

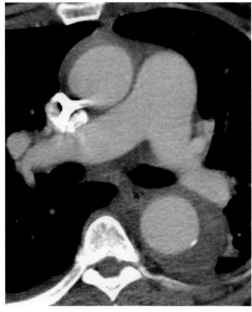

Case 22 Intramural Hematoma

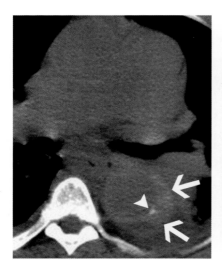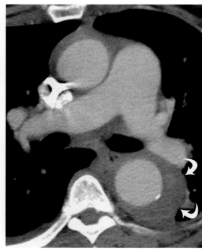

Findings

▶ Location: Descending aorta (50%–80%), ascending aorta
▶ CXR: Frontal view: Nonspecific; displaced intimal calcification
▶ CT:
  ▪ NECT: Circumferential/crescentic hyperdense mural thickening along the aortic wall (arrows), displaced intimal calcification (arrowhead)
  ▪ CTA: No intimal flap; hypodense mural thickening (curved arrows); smoothly marginated, contrast-filled aorta
▶ MR:
  ▪ T1 weighted image (T1WI): No intimal flap, high-signal mural thickening
  ▪ T2 weighted image (T2WI): Intermediate- to high-signal mural thickening
  ▪ T1 + gadolinium (T1+Gad): Low-signal mural thickening with high signal within the aortic lumen

Differential Diagnosis

▶ Thrombosed saccular aortic aneurysm
▶ Aortic pseudoaneurysm
▶ Aortic dissection
▶ Aortitis
▶ Penetrating atherosclerotic ulcer

Teaching Points

▶ Hemorrhage due to rupture of the vasa vasorum within the aortic media, between the intima and adventitia, without an intimal tear
▶ Etiology: Spontaneous rupture of the vaso vasorum, penetrating aortic ulcer, trauma, iatrogenic
▶ Epidemiology: Males = females; elderly patients
▶ Presentation: Acute chest pain; overlaps with aortic dissection
▶ Complications: Aortic dissection (25%–45%), aneurysm (30%–40%), or rupture
▶ <30% may completely reabsorb the hematoma

Management

▶ Same treatment as for aortic dissection

Further Reading

Nienaber CA et al. Intramural hemorrhage of the thoracic aorta. Diagnostic and therapeutic implications. *Circulation*. 1995;92(6):1465–1472.

History

▶ A 63-year-old female presents with back pain

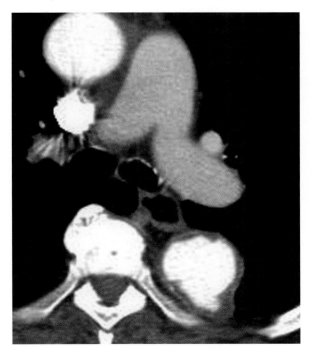

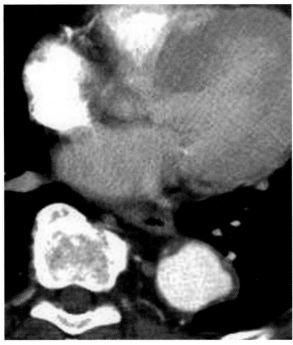

Case 23 Penetrating Atherosclerotic Ulcer

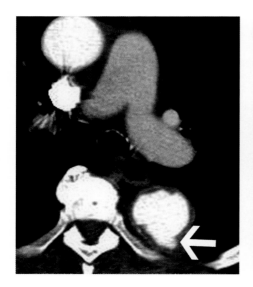 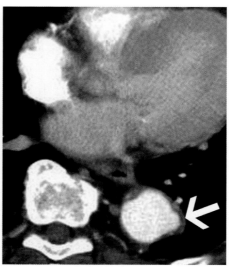

Findings

▶ CTA:
  ■ Focal contrast-filled defect (arrows) within an atherosclerotic lesion of the aortic wall
  ■ Associated with adjacent subintimal hematoma, displaced intimal calcification, aortic wall thickening and enhancement
  ■ Most commonly found in the descending thoracic aorta

Differential Diagnosis

▶ Aortic dissection
▶ Intramural hematoma
▶ Mycotic aortic aneurysm
▶ Aortic pseudoaneurysm

Teaching Points

▶ Also known as *penetrating aortic ulcer*
▶ Ulcerated atherosclerotic lesion penetrating the intima through the elastic lamina and extending into the media
▶ Risk factors: HTN, advanced atherosclerosis, smoking
▶ Epidemiology: Elderly patients
▶ Presentation: Sudden onset of chest or back pain; overlaps with aortic dissection
▶ Complications: Aortic dilatation, aneurysm or rupture, intramural hematoma

Management

▶ Medical management to control hypertension
▶ Surgical or endovascular treatment in certain patients, including those with complications, ascending aorta involvement, and continual pain

Further Reading

Hayashi H et al. Penetrating atherosclerotic ulcer of the aorta: imaging features and disease concept. *Radiographics*. 2000;20(4):995–1005.

Case 24

History

- None

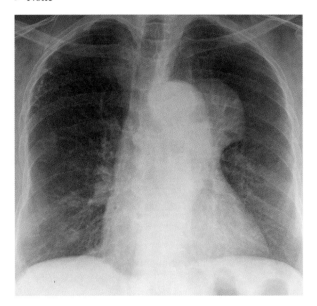

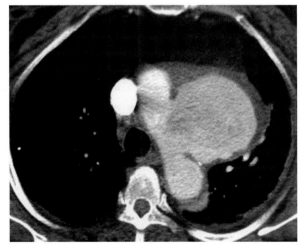

Case 24 Aortic Aneurysm

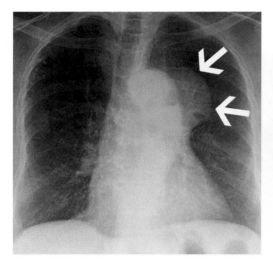 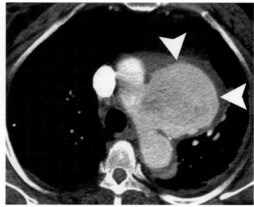

Findings

▶ CXR: Mediastinal mass with a curvilinear rim of calcification (arrows)

▶ CT: Ascending aorta often considered aneurysmal when ≥4 cm; descending thoracic aorta aneurysm ≥3 cm; however, the definition is variable

  ▪ NECT: Dilated aorta, calcification in aneurysm wall, hyperattenuating crescent sign (well-defined crescent of increased attenuation in the mural thrombus, with concern for impending rupture)

  ▪ CTA: Delineates location, extent (local or diffuse), appearance (fusiform or saccular) (arrowheads—*saccular appearance*), and complications; mural thrombus

Differential Diagnosis

▶ Aortic ectasia

▶ Poststenotic aortic dilatation (e.g., aortic stenosis)

▶ Patent ductus arteriosus

Teaching Points

▶ Two types: True (involves all layers) or false/pseudo- (penetration of intima and media, with blood contained by the adventitia or surrounding soft tissue) aneurysm

▶ Etiology: Atherosclerosis, cystic medial necrosis (Marfan syndrome), aortic dissection, trauma (usually pseudoaneurysm), hypertension, aortitis

▶ Epidemiology: Males > females (2–4:1); 3%–4% occur in patients >65 years old

▶ Presentation: Asymptomatic; sometimes acute or chronic chest/back pain

▶ Complications: Aortic dissection or rupture, involvement of major branch vessels, intramural hematoma, erosion into adjacent structures (e.g., aortoenteric fistula)

Management

▶ Surgical or endovascular treatment in patients with symptoms or congenital etiologies; increase in size ≥1 cm/yr; ascending aneurysm >5 cm, descending aneurysm >6 cm

Further Reading
Posniak HV et al. CT of thoracic aortic aneurysms. *Radiographics*. 1990;10(5):839–855.

History

▶ A 40-year-old female present with shortness of breath

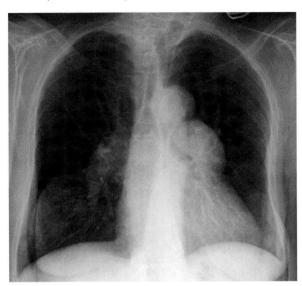

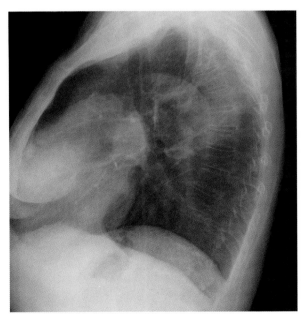

Case 25 Pulmonary Arterial Hypertension

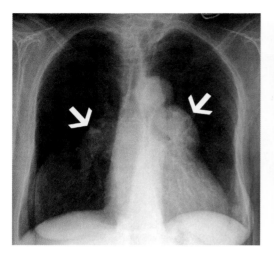 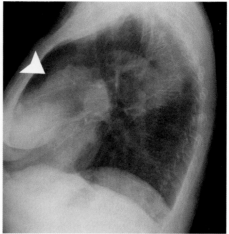

Findings

▶ CXR:
- Frontal view: Dilated central PAs (arrows), convex left PA segment, pruning of peripheral vessels, peripheral oligemia
- Lateral view: RV hypertrophy with filling of the retrosternal clear space (arrowhead)

▶ CT: Geographic ground-glass attenuation (mosaic attenuation) with small-caliber vessels in the underperfused areas, cor pulmonale, atherosclerosis of the PA, diameter of the main PA >3 cm, visible etiology (e.g., chronic thromboembolic disease)

Differential Diagnosis

▶ Hilar adenopathy
▶ Pulmonary artery stenosis
▶ Idiopathic dilation of the pulmonary artery

Teaching Points

▶ Mean pulmonary artery pressure >25 mmHg at rest (>30 mmHg during exercise)
▶ Etiology: Idiopathic (primary), chronic thromboembolic disease (e.g., thrombus, talcosis), sickle cell disease, Eisenmenger physiology (e.g., ventricular septal defect [VSD], atrial septal defect [ASD]), mediastinal fibrosis, connective tissue disease, chronic hypoxia (e.g., chronic obstructive pulmonary disease [COPD], interstitial pulmonary fibrosis [IPF])
▶ Epidemiology: Females > males (3:1) in idiopathic conditions
▶ Presentation: Nonspecific dyspnea
▶ Complications: Right heart failure, pulmonary artery dissection or thrombosis

Management

▶ Treat the underlying pathology
▶ If the condition is idiopathic, medical treatment has limited success but may delay progression of disease, however, it is not curative. Lung transplantation may be necessary.

Further Reading

Frazier AA et al. From the archives of the AFIP: pulmonary vasculature: hypertension and infarction. *Radiographics*. 2000;20(2):491–524.

History

▶ A 36-year-old male with human immunodeficiency virus (HIV) and shortness of breath

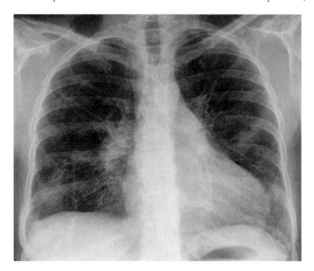

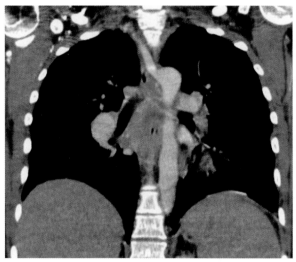

Case 26 Pulmonary Artery Aneurysm

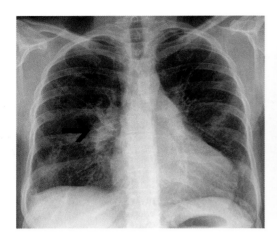 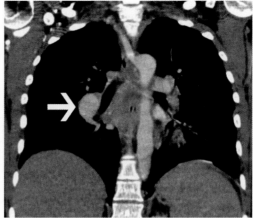

Findings

- ► CXR: Frontal view: Nonspecific hilar enlargement (black arrow) or pulmonary nodule if peripheral
- ► CTA: Focal dilation of a PA (white arrow); enhancement is identical to that of adjacent PAs
  - ▪ If it is a Rasmussen aneurysm: located near the cavitating lesion (due to tuberculosis [TB])

Differential Diagnosis

- ► Hilar adenopathy
- ► Pulmonary arterial hypertension
- ► Pulmonic stenosis with poststenotic dilation (main and left PAs)
- ► Idiopathic dilation of a PA (main PA)
- ► Solitary pulmonary nodule (if peripheral)

Teaching Points

- ► Two types: True (involves all layers) or false/pseudo- (penetration of intima and media with blood contained by the adventitia) aneurysm
- ► Etiology: Iatrogenic (e.g., due to a Swan-Ganz catheter), pulmonary arterial hypertension, vasculitis (e.g., Behçet disease), infection (mycotic), trauma
- ► Presentation: Usually asymptomatic; also hemoptysis, dyspnea
- ► Complications: PA dissection or rupture, pericardial tamponade, thromboembolic disease

Management

- ► Treatment of underlying pathology
- ► Surgical or endovascular treatment in patients with peripheral aneurysm (Swan-Ganz or Rasmussen aneurysm)
- ► Surgical treatment in patients with a central aneurysm

Further Reading

Castañer E et al. Congenital and acquired pulmonary artery anomalies in the adult: radiologic overview. *Radiographics.* 2006;26(2):349–371.

History

▶ A 29-year-old male with a history of TOF repair presents with chest pain

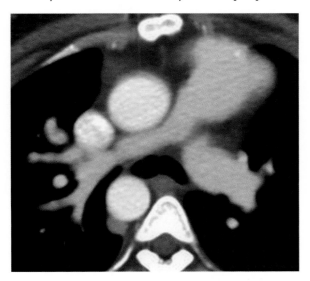

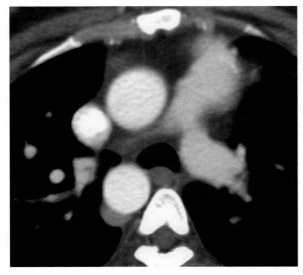

Case 27 Pulmonary Artery Stenosis

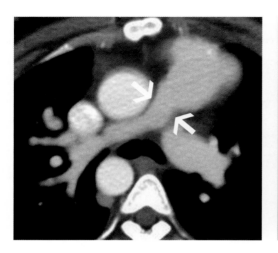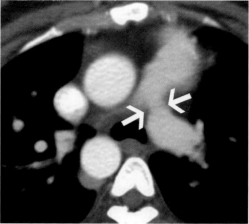

Findings

- CXR:
  - Frontal view: Poststenotic dilatation of the PA distal to narrowing
  - Lateral view: RV hypertrophy with filling of the retrosternal clear space
- CT:
  - NECT: Mosaic attenuation, concentric vascular wall thickening, poststenotic dilatation, RV hypertrophy
  - CTA: Focal or segmental tubular narrowing of the PA (arrows), prominent aortopulmonary collateral vessels on the ipsilateral side if stenosis is severe

Differential Diagnosis

- Pulmonary artery aneurysm/pseudoaneurysm (on CXR)
- Chronic thromboembolic disease

Teaching Points

- Etiology: Chronic thromboembolic disease, fibrosing mediastinitis, mediastinal mass (extrinsic compression), iatrogenic (surgery involving the PA), systemic vasculitis (e.g., Takayasu arteritis, Behçet disease), connective tissue disorders, other syndromes (e.g., Williams syndrome, congenital rubella, Ehlers-Danlos syndrome)
- Associated with TOF, pulmonary atresia
- Presentation: Progressive dyspnea, elevated PA pressure, hemoptysis, cyanosis (tetralogy of Fallot)
- Complications: Pulmonary artery aneurysm, pseudoaneurysm

Management

- Surgical treatment for TOF
- Endovascular treatment (balloon angioplasty ± stent placement) for select patients

Further Readings

Kreutzer J et al. Isolated peripheral pulmonary artery stenoses in the adult. *Circulation.* 1996;93(7):1417–1423.

Pelage JP et al. Pulmonary artery interventions: an overview. *Radiographics.* 2005;25(6):1653–1667.

History

▶ A 29-year-old female with a history of cardiac surgery presents with dyspnea

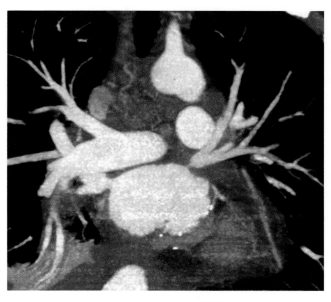

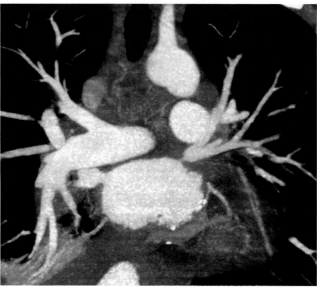

Case 28 Pulmonary Vein Stenosis

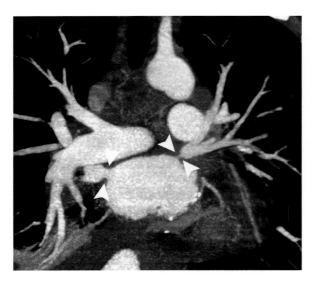

Findings

- CXR: Ipsilateral pulmonary edema (Kerley B lines, pleural effusion)
- CTA/MR: Focal narrowing of the PV (arrowheads), delayed enhancement of the PA and the affected PV
  - Phase-contrast MR: Increased velocity across the narrowing
- X-ray Angiography (XA): Pruning of peripheral arteries, delayed contrast through a narrowed PV

Differential Diagnosis

- PV thrombosis

Teaching Points

- Etiology: Iatrogenic (e.g., radiofrequency catheter ablation for atrial fibrillation, thoracic surgery involving or adjacent to a PV), congenital, mediastinal mass, sarcoidosis, fibrosing medastinitis
- Presentation: Usually asymptomatic; also dyspnea, cough, hemoptysis, pleuritic pain
- Complication: PA hypertension

Management

- Surgical or endovascular treatment (percutaneous balloon angioplasty ± stent placement)

Further Readings

Lacomis JM et al. Multi-detector row CT of the left atrium and pulmonary veins before radio-frequency catheter ablation for atrial fibrillation. *Radiographics.* 2003;23 Spec No:S35–S48; discussion S48–S50.
Latson LA et al. Congenital and acquired pulmonary vein stenosis. *Circulation.* 2007;115(1):103–108.
van Son JA et al. Repair of congenital and acquired pulmonary vein stenosis. *Ann Thorac Surg.* 1995;60(1):144–150.

Part 4

Congenital Heart Disease— Cardiac

History

▶ None

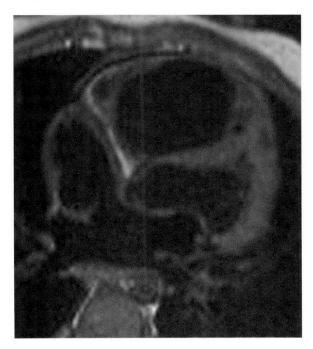

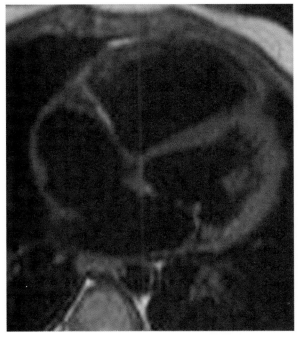

Case 29 Ostium Secundum Atrial Septal Defect

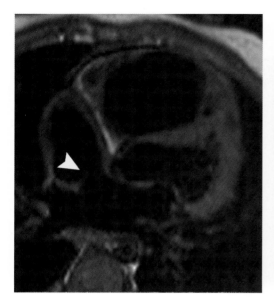 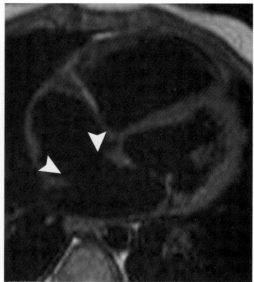

Findings

- ► CXR: Frontal view: Normal to mild cardiomegaly, dilated central and peripheral PAs in adults
- ► CTA/MR: Defect in atrial septum (arrowheads), RA and RV enlargement, normal LA, dilated central PA
  - ■ MR can also evaluate blood flow, including shunt severity, by assessing the ratio of pulmonary to systemic flow

Differential Diagnosis

- ► Other types of ASD (e.g., ostium primum, sinus venosus)
- ► VSD
- ► Pulmonary arterial hypertension

Teaching Points

- ► Defect(s) in the atrial septum of the heart; most common type of ASD (70%)
- ► Isolated or associated with other congenital heart disease
- ► Epidemiology: Females > males (2:1); most common adult congenital heart disease
- ► Presentation: Usually asymptomatic, heart murmurs
- ► Complications: Pulmonary arterial hypertension, paradoxical emboli, atrial arrhythmia

Management

- ► None; small defects may close spontaneously in children
- ► Endovascular (e.g., transcatheter percutaneous closure device) or surgical (e.g., Dacron patch or direct suture closure) treatment

Further Reading

Wang ZJ et al. Cardiovascular shunts: MR imaging evaluation. *Radiographics*. 2003;23 Spec No:S181–S194.

History

▶ None

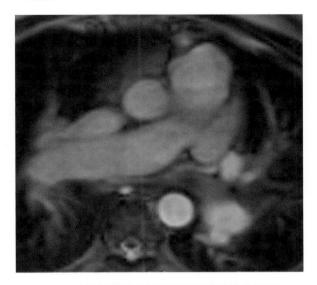

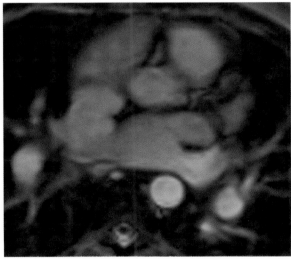

Case 30 Sinus Venosus Atrial Septal Defect

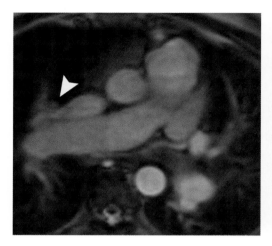 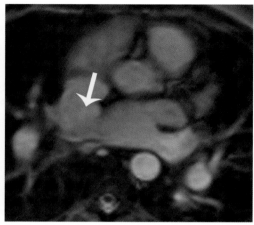

Findings

- ▶ CXR: Frontal view: Normal or dilated central and peripheral PAs, associated PAPVR (the horizontal right upper PV drains into the SVC in PAPVR)
- ▶ CTA/MR: High defect in the atrial septum between the SVC and the LA (arrow), RV enlargement, normal LA, dilated central PA, associated PAPVR (arrowhead)
  - ▪ MR can also evaluate function and flow, including shunt severity, by assessing the ratio of pulmonary to systemic flow

Differential Diagnosis

- ▶ Other types of ASD (e.g., ostium primum, ostium secundum)
- ▶ VSD
- ▶ PAPVR
- ▶ Pulmonary arterial hypertension

Teaching Points

- ▶ Defect(s) in the atrial septum of the heart; unusual type of ASD (10%)
- ▶ Associated with PAPVR (nearly 100%)
- ▶ Presentation: Usually asymptomatic, heart murmurs
- ▶ Complications: Pulmonary arterial hypertension, paradoxical emboli, atrial arrhythmia

Management

- ▶ Surgical treatment using a patch to redirect the right superior PV to the LA effectively closes the ASD and corrects the PAPVR

Further Readings

Kafka H et al. Cardiac MRI and pulmonary MR angiography of sinus venosus defect and partial anomalous pulmonary venous connection in cause of right undiagnosed ventricular enlargement. *AJR Am J Roentgenol*. 2009;192(1):259–266.

Wang ZJ et al. Cardiovascular shunts: MR imaging evaluation. *Radiographics*. 2003;23 Spec No:S181–S194.

History

▸ None

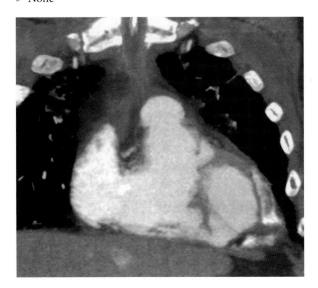

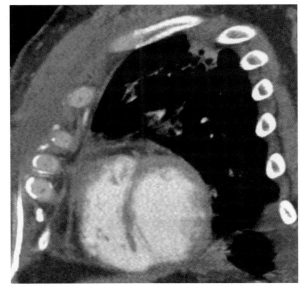

Case 31 Ventricular Septal Defect

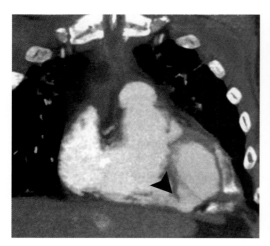
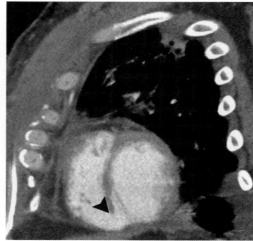

Findings

- ▶ CXR: Frontal view: Cardiomegaly, dilated central and peripheral PAs, left atrial enlargement
- ▶ CTA/MR: Defect in the ventricular septum (arrowheads)
  - ▪ MR can also evaluate blood flow, including shunt severity, by assessing the ratio of pulmonary to systemic flow

Differential Diagnosis

- ▶ Atrioventricular septal defect
- ▶ Patent ductus arteriosus
- ▶ Double-outlet right ventricle

Teaching Points

- ▶ Defect(s) in the ventricular septum; classification based on location and margin (outlet, membranous, trabecular, inlet)
- ▶ Associated with other congenital heart disease (e.g., TOF, truncus arteriosus, double-outlet RV, tricuspid atresia)
- ▶ Epidemiology: Males = females, second most common congenital heart disease
- ▶ Presentations: Asymptomatic with a heart murmur or tachypnea, congestive heart failure, tachycardia, diaphoresis, failure to thrive, depending on the size of the defect
- ▶ Complication: Pulmonary arterial hypertension

Management

- ▶ None; small defects may close spontaneously
- ▶ Medical treatment (e.g., diuretics, afterload reduction) followed by surgical treatment, depending on the type of VSD

Further Reading

Varaprasathan GA et al. Quantification of flow dynamics in congenital heart disease: applications of velocity-encoded cine MR imaging. *Radiographics*. 2002;22(4):895–905.

History

▶ None

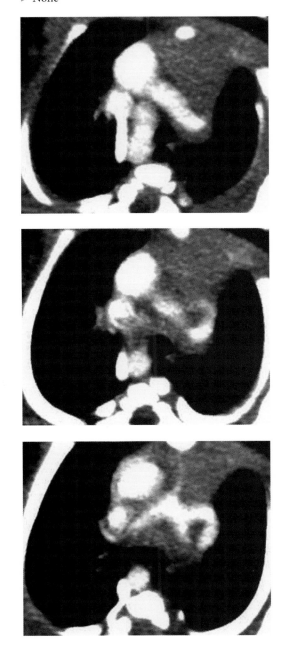

Case 32   Patent Ductus Arteriosus

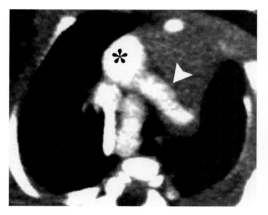 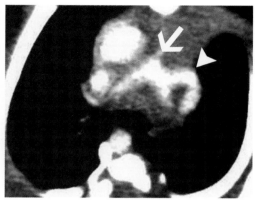

Findings

- ► CXR: Frontal view: Cardiomegaly, dilated central PA, enlarged aortic arch
- ► CTA/MR: Persistent patent prenatal vessel (arrowheads), from the main PA (arrow) to the proximal descending aorta (asterisk), allowing left-to-right shunting

Differential Diagnosis

- ► Other etiologies of left-to-right shunting (e.g., atrioventricular septal defect, VSD, aortopulmonary septal defect)

Teaching Points

- ► With fetal circulation, the ductus allows right-to-left blood flow; postnatally, the increase in oxygen pressure closes the ductus (~18–24 hours), which becomes the ligamentum arteriosum
- ► Associated with prematurity, complex congenital heart disease (e.g., hypoplastic left heart syndrome, preductal aortic coarctation, dextrotransposition of great arteries [D-TGA], pulmonary atresia), persistent fetal circulation (e.g., surfactant deficiency)
- ► Presentation: Asymptomatic, machinery murmur, bounding pulse
- ► Complications: Pulmonary arterial hypertension, Eisenmenger physiology, renal dysfunction

Management

- ► Medical treatment used to close the ductus in premature infants (indomethacin) or to keep the ductus patent in infants with cyanotic heart disease (prostaglandin E1)
- ► Surgical (clipping or ligation) or endovascular (coils) treatment used to close the ductus in mature infants

Further Reading

Goitein O et al. Incidental finding on MDCT of patent ductus arteriosus: use of CT and MRI to assess clinical importance. *AJR Am J Roentgenol*. 2005;184(6):1924–1931.

History

▶ A 23-year-old male with dyspnea on exertion and cyanosis

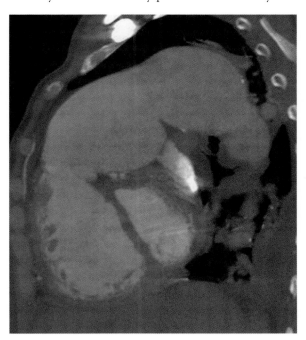

Figure 33-1   Image courtesy of Jean Jeudy, MD (University of Maryland Medical Center, Baltimore, Maryland)

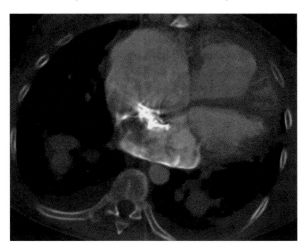

Figure 33-2   Image courtesy of Jean Jeudy, MD (University of Maryland Medical Center, Baltimore, Maryland)

Case 33 Left-to-Right Shunt Reversal—Eisenmenger Physiology

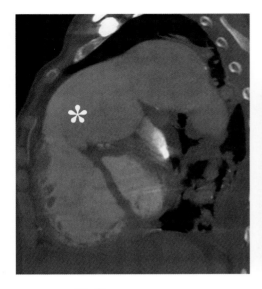
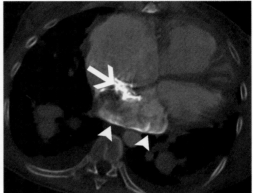

Findings

- ► CXR:
  - Frontal view: Dilated central and peripheral PAs, convex left PA segment, enlarged right heart border due to RA enlargement
  - Lateral view: RV enlargement with filling of the retrosternal clear space
- ► CTA/MR: RA and RV enlargement, cor pulmonale, enlarged main PA (asterisk), associated congenital heart defects (arrow), right-to-left or bidirectional intracardiac shunting (arrowheads)

Differential Diagnosis

- ► Primary pulmonary hypertension
- ► Cyanotic congenital heart disease (e.g., TOF)

Teaching Points

- ► Etiology: Uncorrected congenital heart disease with an intracardiac connection (e.g., ASD, VSD, patent ductus arteriosus [PDA]) eventually results in irreversible pulmonary HTN (>25 mmHg during rest, >30 mmHg during stress) and reversal of the normal left-to-right intracardiac shunt
- ► Presentation: Cyanosis, dyspnea upon exertion, syncope, chest pain, congestive heart failure, dysrhythmia, pulmonary hemorrhage/hemoptysis
- ► Complication: Paradoxical embolus

Management

- ► Medical treatment (e.g., pulmonary vasodilators) can potentially treat the symptoms and delay surgical treatment
- ► Heart-lung transplantation or single or bilateral sequential lung transplantation ± repair of the congenital heart defect are the only curative procedures

Further Reading

Vongpatanasin W et al. The Eisenmenger syndrome in adults. *Ann Intern Med.* 1998;128(9):745–755.

History

▶ None

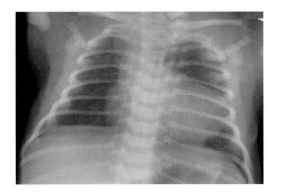

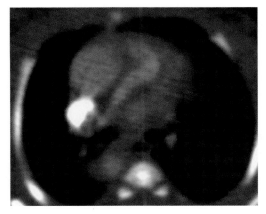

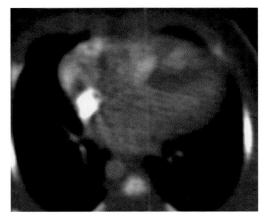

Case 34 Uncorrected Tetralogy of Fallot

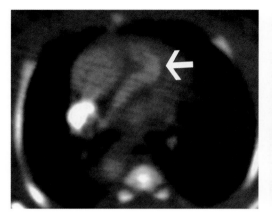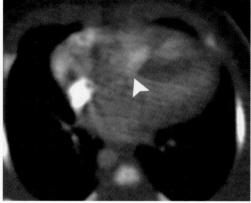

Findings

- ► CXR: Frontal view: "Boot-shaped" heart, pulmonary oligemia
- ► CTA/MR: Four key anatomic features: (1) subvalvular (infundibular) or valvular stenosis of the RVOT (arrow), (2) overriding aorta, (3) subaortic VSD (arrowhead), and (4) RV hypertrophy; prominent collateral vessels
  - ▪ MR can also estimate RV function (e.g., ejection fraction)

Differential Diagnosis

- ► Tricuspid atresia with ASD ± VSD/PDA ± transposition of great arteries (TGA)
- ► Double-outlet RV with pulmonary stenosis
- ► Trilogy of Fallot (RVOT stenosis, RV hypertrophy, ASD)
- ► Pentalogy of Fallot (TOF + ASD)

Teaching Points

- ► Most common cyanotic congenital heart disease
- ► Associated with left PA stenosis, absent pulmonary valve, right aortic arch, malignant anomalous origin of the RCA, scoliosis
- ► Presentation:
  - ▪ Neonates—cyanosis, "tet" spells (bluish skin from crying or feeding)
  - ▪ Children—squatting improves dyspnea on exertion

Management

- ► Surgical treatment (dilation of the RVOT stenosis and closure of the VSD) should be performed to improve the long-term prognosis

Further Reading

Haramati LB et al. MR imaging and CT of vascular anomalies and connections in patients with congenital heart disease: significance in surgical planning. *Radiographics*. 2002;22(2):337–347.

History

▶ None

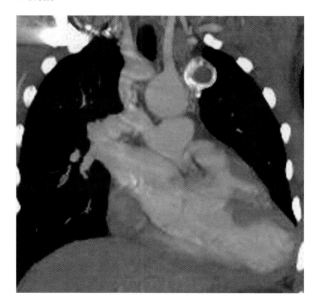

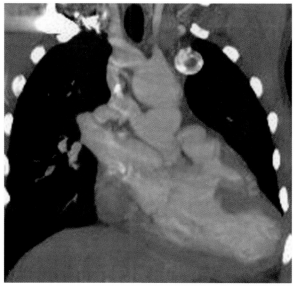

Case 35   Corrected Tetralogy of Fallot

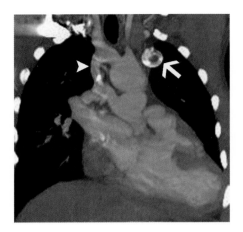

Findings: Two types of repairs

▶ Definitive repair:
- CXR: Lateral view: RV hypertrophy with filling of the retrosternal clear space
- CT: Unenhanced, possibly calcified patch between the overriding aortic annulus and the existing ventricular septum (VSD repair), patch from the RVOT or RA to the distal main PA (RVOT stenosis repair), RV hypertrophy
- MR: T1 + Gad: Delayed ventricular hyperenhancement (fibrosis)

▶ Palliative repair (see below for types):
- CXR: Frontal view: Ipsilateral rib notching, findings of pulmonary HTN
- CTA: Contrast-filled shunt (arrowhead), ± associated findings of TOF
- MR: Tubular flow signal, depending on the type of sequence

Teaching Points

▶ Definitive repair:
- Closure of VSD and enlargement of RVOT stenosis using a patch (± resection of obstructing muscles)
- Complications: Cardiac arrhythmias, pulmonary regurgitation, RV dilatation and dysfunction, PA stenosis, Major Aorto-Pulmonary Collateral Arteries (MAPCA)

▶ Palliative repair:
- Shunts created to increase pulmonary blood flow
  - Blalock-Taussig shunt—redirection of the proximal subclavian artery (ligation of the distal subclavian artery) anastomosing to the ipsilateral PA
  - Modified Blalock-Taussig shunt—synthetic graft connecting the subclavian artery or brachiocephalic trunk to the ipsilateral PA
- Complications: Subclavian artery or graft occlusion (see the arrow in the case), perigraft seroma

Management

▶ Definitive repair is usually performed in early childhood with removal of the palliative shunts
▶ Medical or endovascular treatments for definitive repair complications

Further Reading

Norton KI et al. Cardiac MR imaging assessment following tetralogy of Fallot repair. *Radiographics.* 2006;26(1):197–211.

History

▶ None

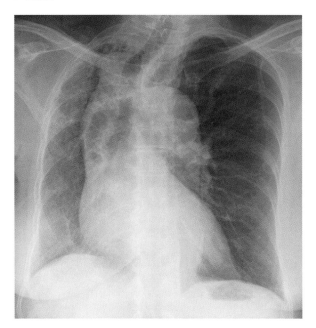

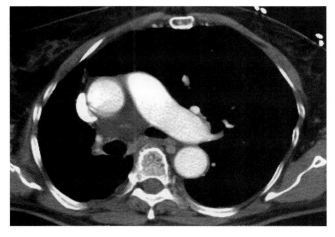

Case 36 Absent Pulmonary Artery

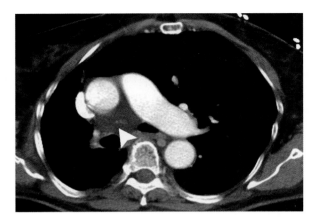

Findings

▶ CXR: Frontal view: Volume loss of ipslateral hemithorax with contralateral lung
hyperinflation, mediastinal shift to the affected side, a peripheral fine reticular pattern,
pleural thickening, rib notching
▶ CT:
  ▪ NECT: Pleural thickening and peripheral fine reticular opacities of the affected
  hemithorax
  ▪ Contrast-enhanced computed tomography (CECT): Complete absence of the proximal
  PA (arrowhead), mediastinal shift to the affected side, enlarged collateral vessels

Differential Diagnosis

▶ Swyer-James syndrome

Teaching Points

▶ During development, only the extrapulmonary PA fails to develop ("absent"), while the
intrapulmonary PAs are normal
▶ Isolated or associated with other congenital heart disease
▶ Presentation: Asymptomatic, dyspnea on exertion, hemoptysis
▶ Complications: Recurrent lung infections, contralateral pulmonary artery stenosis,
contralateral pulmonary hypertension

Management

▶ If detected early, surgical treatment (e.g., aortopulmonary shunt or connecting the affected
PA to the main PA) can be performed

Further Readings

Apostolopoulou SC et al. "Absent" pulmonary artery in one adult and five pediatric patients: imaging,
embryology, and therapeutic implications. *AJR Am J Roentgenol.* 2002;179(5):1253–1260.
Ryu DS et al. HRCT findings of proximal interruption of the right pulmonary artery. *J Thorac Imaging.*
2004;19(3):171–175.

History

▶ None

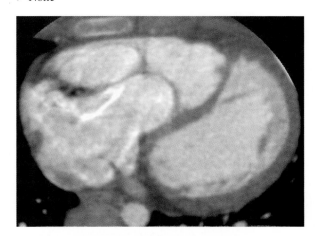

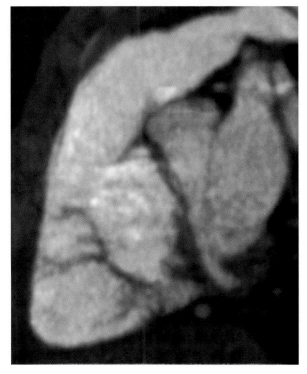

Case 37 Ebstein Anomaly

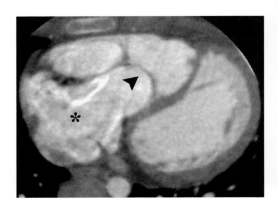 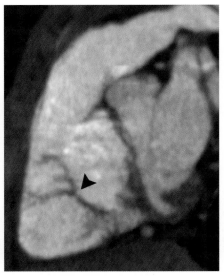

Findings

▶ CXR: Frontal view: "Box-shaped" heart (RA enlargement), decreased pulmonary vascularity
▶ CTA/MR: Downward displacement of the septal and posterior leaflets of the tricuspid valve into the inflow portion of the RV (arrowheads), "atrialized" RV, "sail-like" anterior leaflet, RA enlargement (asterisk), ± associated findings
  ▪ Cine: Retrograde flow during systole (tricuspid regurgitation)

Differential Diagnosis

▶ Large ASD
▶ Pericardial effusion
▶ Tricuspid regurgitation
▶ Uhl anomaly
▶ Arrhythmogenic right ventricular dysplasia (ARVD)
▶ Right-sided obstructive heart disease (e.g., TOF, tricuspid atresia, PA stenosis)

Teaching Points

▶ Associated with patent foramen ovale (PFO), ostium secundum ASD (result in a right-to-left shunt)
▶ Presentation: Asymptomatic or cyanosis
▶ Complications: Fatal atrial arrhythmias, paradoxical embolus

Management

▶ Tricuspid valve replacement (e.g., bioprosthesis) and/or reconstruction (e.g., valvuloplasty) to improve function

Further Reading

Ferguson EC et al. Classic imaging signs of congenital cardiovascular abnormalities. *Radiographics.* 2007;27(5):1323–1334.

History

▸ None

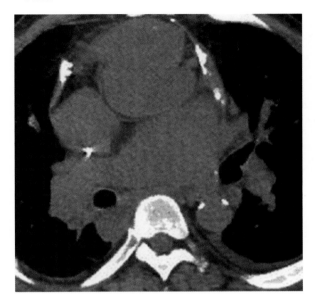

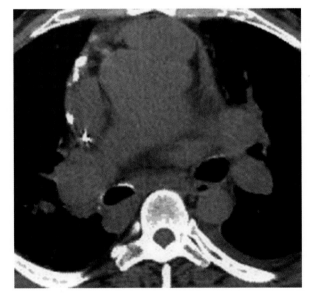

Case 38 Complete (D-) Transposition of Great Arteries

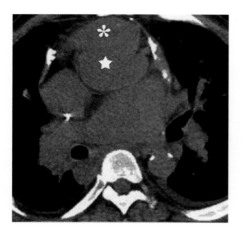

Findings

- ► CXR: Frontal view: Narrowing of the superior mediastinum, "egg on a string" appearance of the cardiovascular silhouette, cardiomegaly, increased pulmonary vascularity
- ► CT/MR: Ventriculoarterial discordance (the PA arises from the LV and connects to the pulmonary circulation, and the aorta arises from the RV and connects to the systemic circulation); the aorta (asterisk) is anterior and to the right of the PA (star)
  - ▪ MR: Can also evaluate function and ventricular volume

Differential Diagnosis

- ► TGA, corrected (L-)

Teaching Points

- ► Most common cyanotic congenital heart defect in neonates, commonly found in patients with diabetic mothers
- ► Isolated or complex, associated with other syndromes or defects
- ► Incompatible with life unless associated with flow admixture (VSD > ASD, PDA)
- ► Also associated with coronary anomalies
- ► Presentation: Severe cyanosis

Management

- ► Medical treatment using prostaglandin E1 to maintain ductus arteriosus patency
- ► Depending on the timing of surgical repair and the degree of ASD, emergent balloon atrial septostomy can be done to improve atrial shunting and mixing (Rashkind operation)
- ► If the neonate is <2–4 weeks old and the coronary arteries can be transplanted, an arterial switch operation (Jatene) can be done to achieve ventriculoarterial concordance
- ► If the Jatene operation cannot be performed, a baffle, made of either right atrial wall/atrial septal tissue (Senning) or pericardium/synthetic material (Mustard), can be formed within the atria in order to reroute the blood flow

Further Readings

Leschka S et al. Pre- and postoperative evaluation of congenital heart disease in children and adults with 64-section CT. *Radiographics.* 2007;27(3):829–846.

Warnes CA et al. Transposition of the great arteries. *Circulation.* 2006;114(24):2699–2709.

History

▸ None

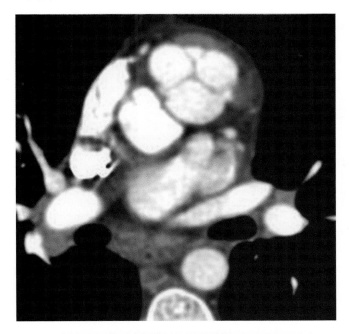

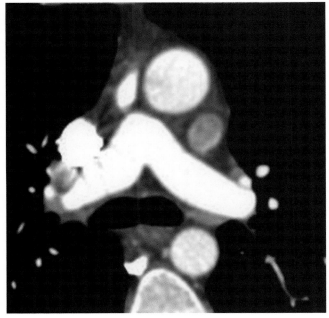

Case 39   Corrected (L-) Transposition of Great Arteries

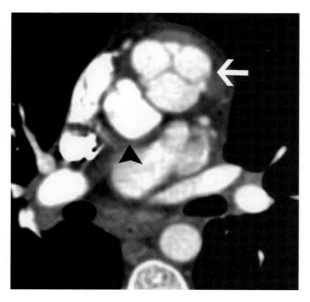

Findings

- ▶ CXR: Frontal view: Straight upper left heart border
- ▶ CTA/MR: Atrioventricular and ventriculoarterial discordance (the LV arises from the RA and connects to the PA and the pulmonary circulation, and the RV arises from the LA and connects to the aorta and the systemic circulation); the PA (arrowhead) is posterior and to the right of the aorta (arrow)
  - ▪ MR: Can evaluate the function of RV in sustaining systemic pressure

Differential Diagnosis

- ▶ TGA, complete (D-)

Teaching Points

- ▶ Associated with VSD > left ventricular outflow tract (LVOT) (subpulmonary) obstruction, Ebstein anomaly, conduction disturbances
- ▶ Presentation: Depends on associated abnormalities
- ▶ Complications: Aortic valve dysfunction and left-sided RV failure due to sustained exposure to the systemic circulation

Management

- ▶ Pacemaker insertion to control conduction disturbances
- ▶ Double-switch procedure—venous switch (Senning) and ventricular (Rastelli) or arterial switch—is performed to prevent late RV failure

Further Readings

Chang DS et al. Congenitally corrected transposition of the great arteries: imaging with 16-MDCT. *AJR Am J Roentgenol.* 2007;188(5):W428–W430.
Warnes CA et al. Transposition of the great arteries. *Circulation.* 2006;114(24):2699–2709.

History

▶ None

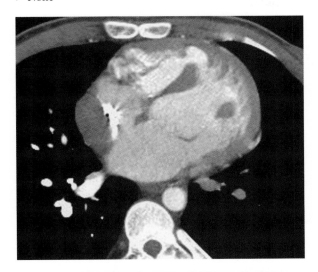

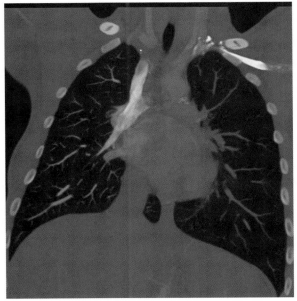

Case 40 Tricuspid Atresia

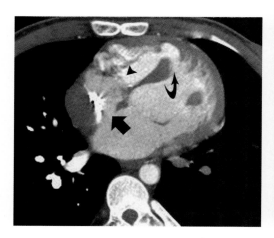
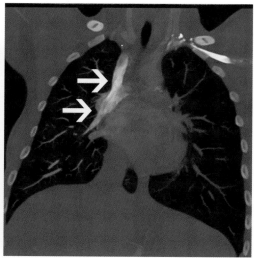

Findings

- ► CXR: Frontal view: Normal to cardiomegaly
- ► CTA/MR: Absence of the tricuspid valve and the inlet portion of the RV (black arrowhead), ASD (block arrow), VSD (curved arrow), other associated findings ± postsurgical changes such as the SVC connecting to the PA (white arrows)

Differential Diagnosis

- ► TGA
- ► TOF
- ► Ebstein anomaly

Teaching Points

- ► Incompatible with life unless associated with ASD or PDA ± VSD (or D-TGA)
- ► Also associated with PA stenosis/atresia
- ► Presentation: Cyanosis, congestive heart failure

Management

- ► Medical (e.g., prostaglandin E1) to maintain PDA patency prior to surgery
- ► Surgical treatment to maintain PA flow
  - ▪ Atrial septostomy to allow adequate interatrial shunting
  - ▪ Modified Blalock-Taussig shunt—synthetic graft connecting the subclavian artery or brachiocephalic trunk to the ipsilateral PA
  - ▪ Total cavopulmonary connection—bidirectional Glenn and Fontan completion procedures that connect the SVC and IVC, respectively, to the PA

Further Reading

Siegel MJ et al. MDCT of postoperative anatomy and complications in adults with cyanotic heart disease. *AJR Am J Roentgenol.* 2005;184(1):241–247.

History

▶ None

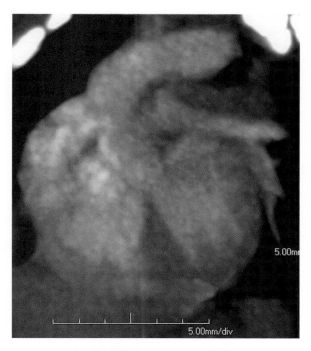

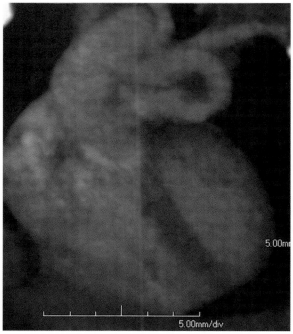

Case 41 Truncus Arteriosus

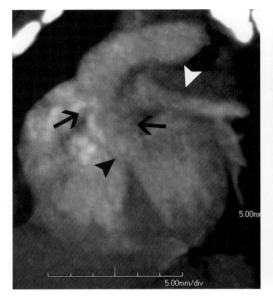
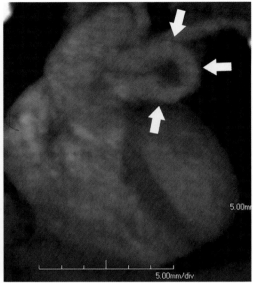

Findings

▶ CXR: Frontal view: Cardiomegaly, increased pulmonary vascularity, narrow mediastinum (thymic agenesis), right aortic arch
▶ CTA/MR:
  ▪ A common arterial trunk (black arrows) arises from both ventricles and becomes the aorta, PAs (white arrowhead), and coronaries
  ▪ VSD (black arrowhead), PDA (white arrows), other associated findings, postoperative complications

Differential Diagnosis

▶ TGA
▶ Aortopulmonary window
▶ Atrioventricular (AV) canal defect

Teaching Points

▶ Classification (Collett/Edwards or Van Praagh) depends on the precise location of the PAs arising from the common arterial trunk
▶ Associated with right aortic arch with mirror imaging (30%–40%), VSD, PDA, DiGeorge anomaly (including absent thymus and parathyroid glands)
▶ Presentation: Congestive heart failure or cyanosis
▶ Complications: Truncal valve regurgitation, postoperative conditions (e.g., conduit stenosis, anastomotic pseudoaneurysm)

Management

▶ Surgical treatment by closure of the VSD and placement (± revisions) of a conduit between the RV and PA

Further Reading

Donnelly LF et al. MR imaging of conotruncal abnormalities. *AJR Am J Roentgenol*. 1996;166(4): 925–928.

History

▶ None

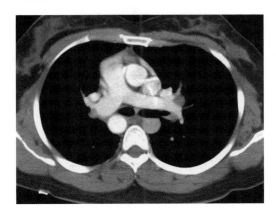

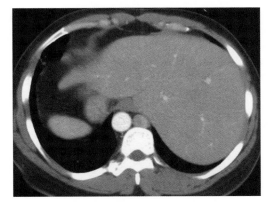

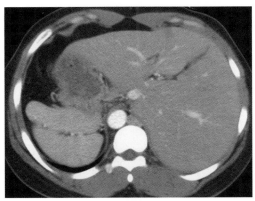

Case 42 Heterotaxy Syndrome

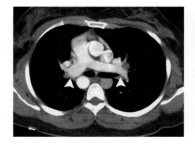 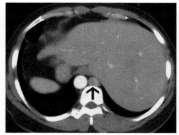 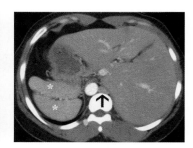

Findings

▶ Two types:
  - Asplenia (also called *double right-sidedness, right isomerism,* and *Ivemark syndrome*)
    - Both lungs have three lobes and eparterial bronchi
    - Associated with atrioventricular septal defect, univentricular heart, TGA, total anomalous pulmonary venous return (TAPVR) (>80%)
  - Polysplenia (also called *double left-sidedness, left isomerism*)
    - Both lungs have two lobes and hyparterial bronchi (arrowheads)
    - Associated with azygous-hemiazygous continuation of the IVC (>70%) (arrows), PAPVR, ASD, atrioventricular septal defect
    - Multilobed spleen (asterisks) or multiple spleens are on the same side as the stomach
▶ Variable cardiac apex (levo-, meso-, or dextrocardia), variable gastric position, centrally located liver, bowel malposition (e.g., midgut volvulus)

Differential Diagnosis

▶ Mislabeled film (CXR)
▶ Situs inversus
▶ Abdominal situs solitus with dextrocardia
▶ Abdominal situs inversus with levocardia
▶ Dextroversion of the heart

Teaching Points

▶ Also known as *situs ambiguous*—disordered organ arrangement in the chest or abdomen, unlike the orderly arrangements in situs solitus or situs inversus
▶ Asplenia: Epidemiology: Male > female; first-year mortality ≤80%; presentation: severe cyanosis
▶ Polysplenia: Epidemiology: Female > male; first-year mortality ≤60%; presentation: variable, asymptomatic (rare) to congestive heart failure

Management

▶ Surgical treatment of cardiac anomalies
▶ Asplenia: Prophylactic antibiotics and pneumococcal vaccination

Further Readings

Applegate KE et al. Situs revisited: imaging of the heterotaxy syndrome. *Radiographics.* 1999;19(4): 837–852.

Fulcher AS et al. Abdominal manifestations of situs anomalies in adults. *Radiographics.* 2002;22(6):1439–1456.

History

▶ None

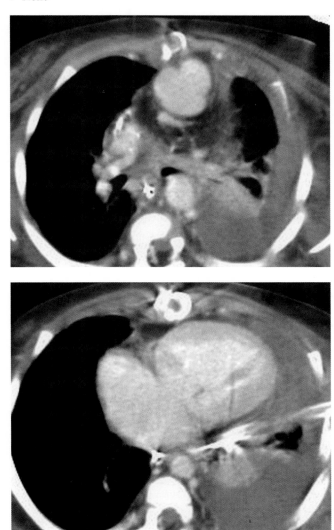

Case 43 Hypoplastic Left Heart Syndrome

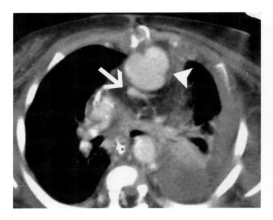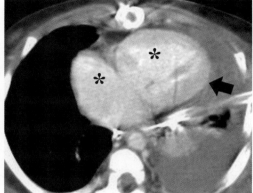

Findings

- ▶ CXR: Frontal view: Cardiomegaly or unusual cardiac silhouette, pulmonary edema (pulmonary venous hypertension), narrow mediastinum (thymic atrophy)
- ▶ CTA/MR: Small LV (block arrow) and aorta (arrow), dilated right cardiac chambers (asterisks) and main PA (arrowhead), associated findings, such as PDA, and postoperative changes
  - ▪ MR can also evaluate function and flow

Differential Diagnosis

- ▶ Aortic stenosis
- ▶ Coarctation of the aorta
- ▶ Interrupted aortic arch

Teaching Points

- ▶ Wide spectrum of cardiac malformations, including hypoplasia/atresia of the aortic and mitral valves and hypoplasia of the LV and ascending aorta
- ▶ PDA is required for early survival; right-to-left blood flow through the PDA to the systemic circulation in systole; left-to-right blood flow through the PDA and retrograde through the ascending aorta to perfuse the cerebral and coronary arteries during diastole
- ▶ Associated with pre- and postductal coarctation of the aorta, PDA, PFO, VSD, double-outlet RV, endocardial fibroelastosis
- ▶ Epidemiology: Males > females (2:1), 0.2/1000 live births; if untreated, causes 25% of all neonatal cardiac deaths
- ▶ Presentation: Cyanosis, congestive heart failure, cardiogenic shock
- ▶ Complications: Right heart failure, tricuspid regurgitation

Management

- ▶ Medical treatment (prostaglandin E1) to keep the ductus patent prior to surgery
- ▶ Palliative surgical treatment (three stages—Norwood, hemi-Fontan or bidirectional Glenn, and Fontan procedures) or cardiac transplantation is required; otherwise, the condition is lethal

Further Reading

Bardo DM et al. Hypoplastic left heart syndrome. *Radiographics*. 2001;21(3):705–717.

Part 5

Ischemic Heart Disease—Coronary Artery Disease

History

▶ None

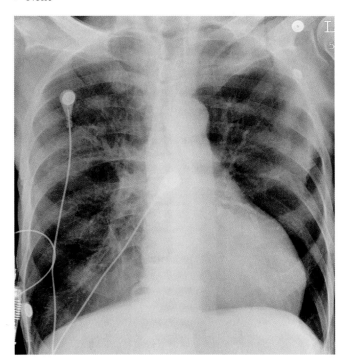

Case 44 Coronary Artery Calcification

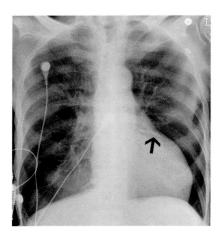

Findings

- ► CXR: "Tram-track" appearance
  - ▪ Visible coronary artery calcification (CAC) on CXR is strongly associated with significant stenosis
- ► CT:
  - ▪ Electron beam computed tomography (EBCT)/NECT: High-density linear or punctate high-density lining of the lumen of the coronary arteries; used for coronary artery calcium scoring (*See Case 45: Coronary Artery Calcium Scoring*)
  - ▪ CECT: CAC may be somewhat obscured by contrast; soft plaque is visible
  - ▪ Overall, more able than CXR to detect calcium

Differential Diagnosis

- ► Pericardial calcification
- ► Myocardial calcification
- ► Valvular calcification

Teaching Points

- ► CAC is a marker of atherosclerotic coronary artery disease (CAD), the leading cause of death in developed countries
  - ▪ Direct relationship with stenosis, total plaque burden, and myocardial infarction (MI)
  - ▪ Relationship is marked in younger patients
- ► Risk factors: hypertension, diabetes mellitus (DM), smoking, hypercholesterolemia, obesity and a sedentary lifestyle, family history
- ► Associated with MI, cardiovascular accident (CVA), renal disease, PVD
- ► Epidemiology: Males (usually >45 years old) > females (usually >55 years old)
- ► Presentation: Asymptomatic to angina, shortness of breath

Management

- ► Initially, lifestyle modifications with medical treatment (e.g., statins) if indicated
- ► Endovascular (percutaneous coronary intervention [PCI]) or surgical (CABG) treatment if associated with advanced disease

Further Reading

Thompson BH et al. Imaging of coronary calcification by computed tomography. *J Magn Reson Imaging.* 2004;19(6):720–733.

History

▶ None

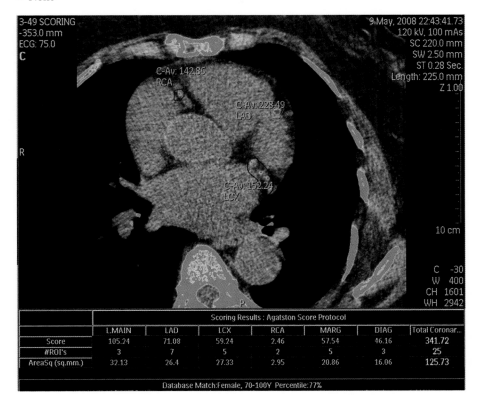

	L.MAIN	LAD	LCX	RCA	MARG	DIAG	Total Coronar...
Scoring Results : Agatston Score Protocol							
Score	105.24	71.08	59.24	2.46	57.54	46.16	341.72
#ROI's	3	7	5	2	5	3	25
AreaSq (sq.mm.)	32.13	26.4	27.33	2.95	20.86	16.06	125.73

Database Match:Female, 70-100Y Percentile:77%

Case 45 Coronary Artery Calcium Scoring

			Scoring Results : Agatston Score Protocol				
	L.MAIN	LAD	LCX	RCA	MARG	DIAG	Total Coronar...
Score	105.24	71.08	59.24	2.46	57.54	46.16	**341.72**
#ROI's	3	7	5	2	5	3	**25**
AreaSq (sq.mm.)	32.13	26.4	27.33	2.95	20.86	16.06	**125.73**
Database Match:Female, 70–100Y Percentile:77%							

Findings

► Provides quantitative evaluation of the extent of the total coronary atherosclerotic plaque burden (circle), not the severity of lumen narrowing
  ■ Used for risk assessment (e.g., a score ≥400 is associated with an increased risk of MI and cardiac death)
► Regions of interest (ROI) are drawn around the CAC for accurate calcium scoring
► EBCT: better temporal resolution, longer experience, largely abandoned
► NECT: better signal-to-noise ratio, wider availability

Teaching Points

► Three methods
  ■ Agatston score: Most common
    ◆ Based on summing the CT values and density (threshold >130 HU) of all CACs
    ◆ Databases that compare the patient's calcium score to the scores of individuals of similar age and the same gender (percentiles) are commonly based on this method
    ◆ Score <10, minimal; 11–99, moderate; 100–400, increased; >400, extensive calcifications
    ◆ Limited by nonlinearity with the amount of calcium
  ■ Volume score: More reproducible
    ◆ Based on the number of voxels above a threshold (typically >130 HU)
    ◆ Limited by partial volume averaging
  ■ Calcium mass score: True physical measure of CAC; reproducible by different CT scanners
    ◆ Calibrated based on the known density of hydroxyapatite in proportion to the number of CACs on the CT images
  ■ Males develop calcifications 10–15 years prior to females
  ■ In asymptomatic individuals, calcifications are commonly seen in males >55 years old and in females >65 years old

Management

► High scores support a more intensive effort to reduce risk factors (e.g., improved diet, increased exercise, smoking cessation) ± additional diagnostic procedures

Further Reading

Hoffmann U et al. Cardiology patient page. Use of new imaging techniques to screen for coronary artery disease. *Circulation.* 2003;108(8):e50–e53.

History

▶ None

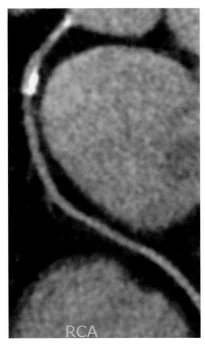

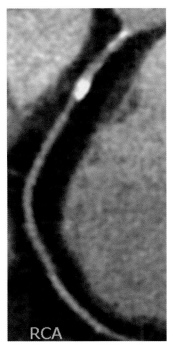

Case 46 Right Coronary Artery Stenosis

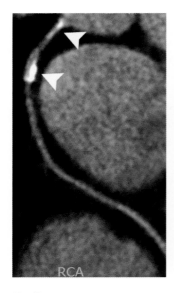 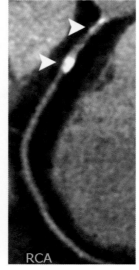

Findings

- ► CTA:
  - ▪ Calcified (arrowheads) and/or noncalcified atherosclerotic plaques, luminal narrowing or occlusion
  - ▪ ≥70% narrowing is considered hemodynamically significant
  - ▪ Best visualized in maximum intensity projection (MIP) and curved multiplanar reconstruction (MPR) images
- ► MR:
  - ▪ Magnetic resonance angiography (MRA): Focal decrease in signal intensity; less sensitive than CTA
  - ▪ Steady-state free precession (SSFP): Inferior/inferoseptal LV wall hypo-/a-/dyskinesis
  - ▪ First-pass perfusion (FPP): Inferior/inferoseptal LV wall defect
  - ▪ Delayed contrast enhancement (CE): Hyperenhancement of nonviable myocardium
- ► XA: Gold standard, findings similar to those of CTA, can assess collateral vessels

Differential Diagnosis

- ► Coronary spasm

Teaching Points

- ► Presentations: Angina, nausea, vomiting or other gastrointestinal (GI) symptoms, bradycardia
- ► Complication: Inferior/inferoseptal LV wall infarction

Management

- ► Medical treatment (e.g., nitrates, β-blockers) for symptomatic relief
- ► Endovascular (e.g., angioplasty) or surgical (e.g., CABG) treatment for coronary revascularization

Further Readings

Achenbach S. Computed tomography coronary angiography. *J Am Coll Cardiol.* 2006;48(10):1919–1928.

Zhang S et al. MDCT in assessing the degree of stenosis caused by calcified coronary artery plaques. *AJR Am J Roentgenol.* 2008;191(6):1676–1683.

History

▸ An 81-year-old male presents with unstable angina

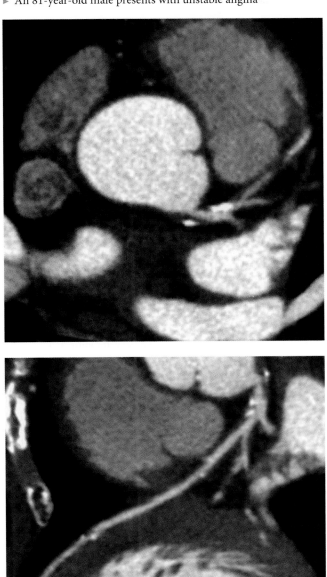

Case 47 Left Main Coronary Artery Stenosis

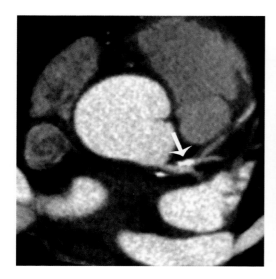 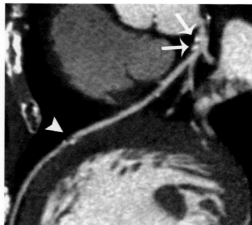

Findings

▶ CTA:
  ▪ Calcified (arrows) and/or noncalcified atherosclerotic plaques, luminal narrowing or occlusion, most commonly at the middle to distal portion
  ▪ >50% narrowing is considered hemodynamically significant
  ▪ Axial images are crucial; best visualized completely in MIP and curved MPR images

▶ MR:
  ▪ MRA: Focal decrease in signal intensity; less sensitive than CTA
  ▪ SSFP: Anterior and lateral LV wall hypo-/a-/dyskinesis
  ▪ FPP: Anterior and lateral LV wall defects
  ▪ Delayed CE: Hyperenhancement of nonviable myocardium

▶ XA: Gold standard, findings similar to those of CTA

Differential Diagnosis

▶ Coronary spasm
▶ Coronary dissection

Teaching Points

▶ 50%–70% narrowing = 66% 3-year survival; >70% narrowing = 41% 3-year survival
▶ Etiology: Atherosclerosis, syphilis, giant cell arteritis, Takayasu arteritis, trauma
▶ Often associated with narrowing in other vessels (80%), such as the LAD (arrowhead)
▶ Presentation: Asymptomatic, unstable or crescendo angina, electrocardiographic (ECG) changes (ST-segment depression and T-wave inversion)
▶ Complication: Heart failure, anterior and lateral LV wall infarction, sudden death

Management

▶ Evolving; CABG is currently the treatment of choice

Further Reading

Taggart DP et al. Revascularization for unprotected left main stem coronary artery stenosis stenting or surgery. *J Am Coll Cardiol.* 2008;51(9):885–892.

History

▶ None

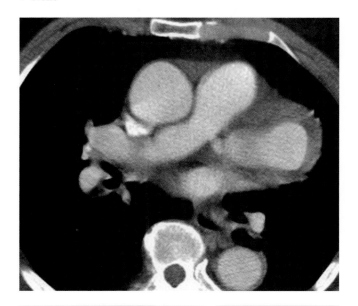

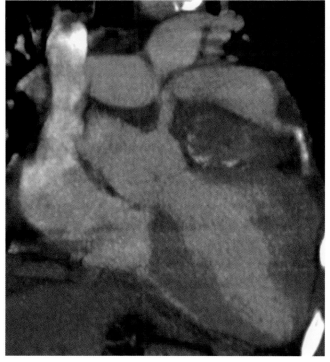

Case 48 Coronary Artery Aneurysm

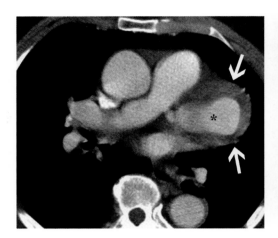 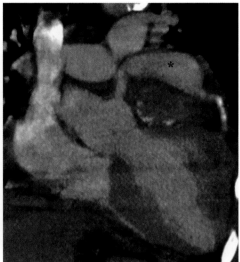

Findings

- ► CTA/MR:
    - Fusiform (asterisks) or saccular, solitary or multiple, dilatation of coronary artery segments (diameter >1.5 times that of the normal adjacent artery segment)
    - Can be thrombosed (arrows) and/or calcified (typically not seen in MR)
    - Most common in the RCA, followed by the LAD coronary artery

Differential Diagnosis

- ► Coronary fistula
- ► CABG aneurysm
- ► Pseudoaneurysm of the ascending aorta or pulmonary trunk
- ► Cardiac or pericardial neoplasm
- ► Thymoma

Teaching Points

- ► Etiology: Kawasaki disease (most common worldwide), atherosclerosis (most common in the United States), mycotic-embolic disease, congenital, trauma, iatrogenic (e.g., PCI), connective tissue disease (e.g., systemic lupus erythematosus, polyarteritis nodosa)
- ► Associated with CAD
- ► Epidemiology: Seen incidentally in up to 4.9% of all coronary angiography cases
- ► Presentation: Asymptomatic, angina, congestive heart failure
- ► Complication: Spontaneous coronary artery dissection

Management

- ► Medical treatment (anticoagulants and antiplatelets) is first-line therapy
- ► If medical treatment fails or there is concomitant CAD, CABG or PCI with stent placement should be considered

Further Reading

Murthy PA et al. MDCT of coronary artery aneurysms. *AJR Am J Roentgenol.* 2005;184(3) (suppl):S19–S20.

History

► None

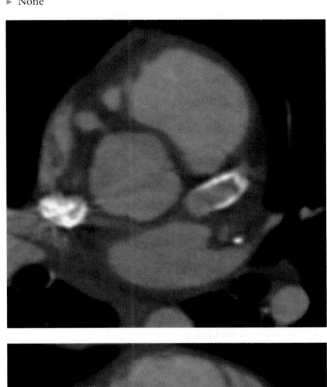

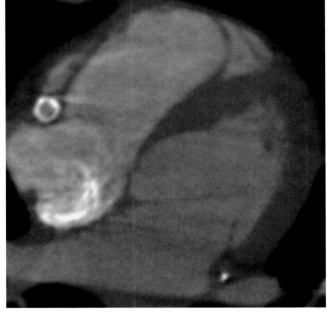

Case 49 Kawasaki Disease

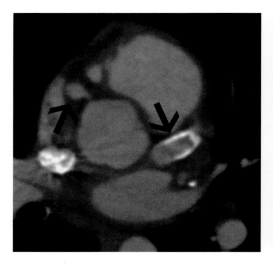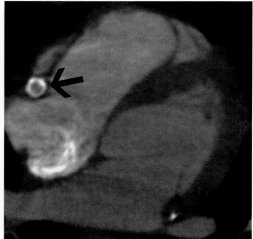

Findings

- ▶ CTA/MR:
  - ▪ Multiple fusiform and saccular dilatations (arrows) and narrowing of coronary and other arteries
  - ▪ Can be thrombosed and/or calcified (calcification often is not seen on MR)
  - ▪ MR can also assess wall motion and function

Differential Diagnosis

- ▶ Other causes of coronary artery aneurysm(s) (e.g., systemic lupus erythematosus, polyarteritis nodosa)
- ▶ Coronary fistula
- ▶ CABG aneurysms

Teaching Points

- ▶ Vasculitis of childhood (medium to large arteries) with multisystem involvement and characteristic progression
- ▶ Epidemiology: Affects mainly Asians; males > females (5:1); two peak periods of incidence (6 months to 2 years old and 5 years old)
- ▶ Presentation: Fever, nonexudative conjunctivitis, erythema of the lips and oral mucosa, skin rash, cervical lymphadenopathy, skin desquamation, elevated C-reactive protein, thrombocytosis
- ▶ Complications: Aneurysmal rupture, cardiac arrhythmia, MI

Management

- ▶ Usually self-limiting; early treatment with intravenous gamma globulin, aspirin
- ▶ CABG is recommended for giant or multiple coronary artery aneurysms or significant stenosis

Further Reading

Mavrogeni S et al. How to image Kawasaki disease: a validation of different imaging techniques. *Int J Cardiol.* 2008;124(1):27–31.

Part 6

Ischemic Heart Disease—Myocardial

History

▸ A 54-year-old male presents with dyspnea and acute chest pain

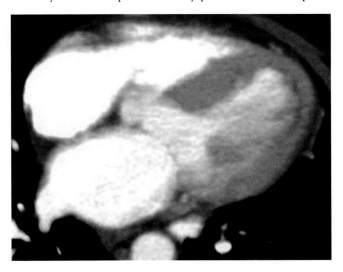

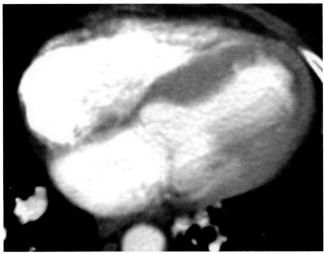

Case 50 Acute Myocardial Infarction

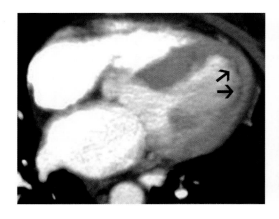 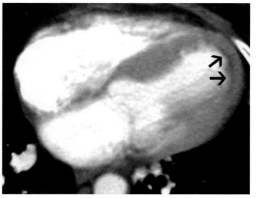

Findings

- ► CXR: Normal to acute pulmonary edema
- ► CTA: Noncalcified coronary artery filling defect, diminished transmural or subendocardial (arrows) enhancement (perfusion) of the affected wall, reduced wall function (contractility), no wall thinning, calcification, or fatty changes
- ► MR:
  - ▪ T2WI: Increased signal intensity (myocardial edema) in affected and surrounding myocardium
  - ▪ SSFP: Regional wall hypo-/a-/dyskinesis
  - ▪ FPP: Reduced perfusion of the regional wall
  - ▪ Delayed CE: Hyperenhancement of the infarcted myocardium

Differential Diagnosis

- ► Chronic MI
- ► Myocarditis
- ► Coronary spasm

Teaching Points

- ► Presentation: Unstable angina, dyspnea, changes on serial ECG, rise and fall of serum cardiac markers (e.g., troponin, creatine kinase)
- ► Complications include ventricular aneurysm or pseudoaneurysm, ventricular septal rupture, pericarditis

Management

- ► Rapid medical therapy (morphine, oxygen, nitrates, aspirin, β-blockers, anticoagulants, additional antiplatelets) and PCI ± stent placement are the mainstay of acute MI treatment

Further Reading

Hoffmann U et al. Cardiac CT in emergency department patients with acute chest pain. *Radiographics*. 2006;26(4):963–978.

History

▶ None

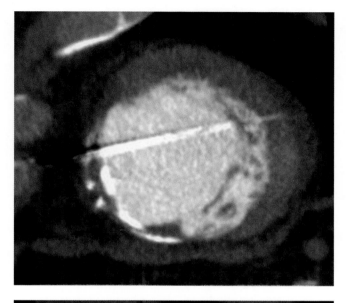

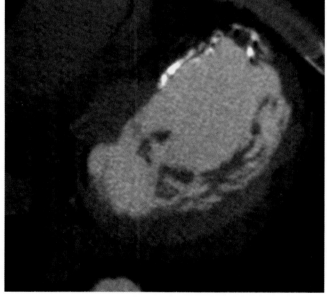

Case 51 Chronic Myocardial Infarction

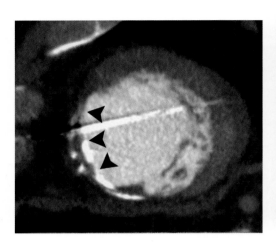 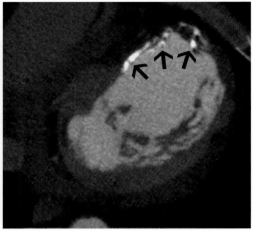

Findings

- ► CXR: Cardiomegaly, myocardial calcification
- ► CTA: Coronary artery filling defect, reduced wall function (contractility), possible myocardial thinning (arrowheads), linear fatty changes or calcifications (arrows) of subendocardial ± transmural myocardium, enlarged LV ± LA
- ► MR:
  - ▪ T2WI: No increased signal intensity in the affected myocardium
  - ▪ SSFP: Regional wall hypo-/a-/dyskinesis
  - ▪ FPP: Reduced perfusion of the regional wall
  - ▪ Delayed CE: Hyperenhancement of nonviable subendocardial ± transmural myocardium

Differential Diagnosis

- ► Acute MI
- ► Nonischemic CM
- ► Endocardial fibroelastosis
- ► ARVD
- ► Constrictive pericarditis

Teaching Points

- ► Associated with LV remodeling with dilatation of the LV cavity
- ► Complications: Mural thrombus, ischemic cardiomyopathy (CM), mitral valve regurgitation, ventricular aneurysm or pseudoaneurysm

Management

- ► Medical therapy (e.g., angiotensin converting enzyme [ACE] inhibitors, aspirin) to reduce ventricular remodeling and prevent additional MI

Further Reading

Cury RC et al. Comprehensive assessment of myocardial perfusion defects, regional wall motion, and left ventricular function by using 64-section multidetector CT. *Radiology*. 2008;248(2):466–475.

History

▸ None

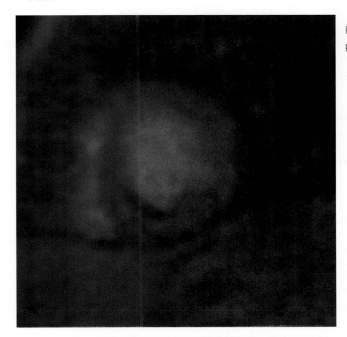

Figure 52-1   First-pass perfusion

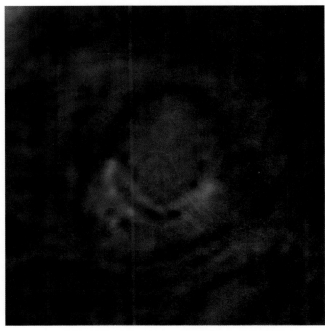

Figure 52-2   Delayed contrast enhancement

Case 52 Microvascular Obstruction

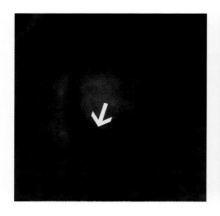 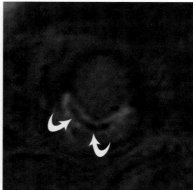

Findings

- MR:
    - T2WI: Increased signal intensity (myocardial edema) in the affected wall
    - FFP: Hypoenhanced or "no-reflow" zone of myocardium (arrow)
    - Delayed CE: Persistent central hypoenhanced zone (core of the myocardial necrosis) with a surrounding zone of delayed enhancement (curved arrows)
        - Most important determinant of functional outcomes—larger infarcts produce worse indices of LV remodeling and significantly lower improvement in LV function over time

Differential Diagnosis

- Acute MI with reperfusion
- Chronic MI
- Stunned myocardium
- Myocarditis
- Vasculitis
- Nonischemic CM (e.g., restrictive CM, dilated CM)
- ARVD

Teaching Points

- Microvascular obstruction is the lack of adequate tissue perfusion within the myocardium from an acute MI, even after restoration of epicardial (coronary) blood flow
- Etiology: Myocardial ischemia-reperfusion injury, distal microembolization from recent PCI or thrombolysis
- Associated with a poor prognosis; the size of the hypoenhanced zones predicts future cardiovascular complications (45% compared to 9%)
- Presentation: Asymptomatic, angina, hemodynamically unstable, conduction changes
- Complications: congestive heart failure (CHF), recurrent infarction, chest pain

Management

- No proven treatment; early revascularization (e.g., a glycoprotein IIb/IIIa receptor inhibitor) or preventive methods (e.g., an embolic protection device) are helpful

Further Readings

Jaffe R et al. Microvascular obstruction and the no-reflow phenomenon after percutaneous coronary intervention. *Circulation*. 2008;117(24):3152–3156.

Nijveldt R et al. Assessment of microvascular obstruction and prediction of short-term remodeling after acute myocardial infarction: cardiac MR imaging study. *Radiology*. 2009;250(2):363–370.

Pineda V et al. No-reflow phenomenon in cardiac MRI: diagnosis and clinical implications. *AJR Am J Roentgenol*. 2008;191(1):73–79.

Reeder SB et al. Advanced cardiac MR imaging of ischemic heart disease. *Radiographics*. 2001;21(4):1047–1074.

History

▶ A 50-year-old male with LV anterior wall dyskinesis on echocardiography

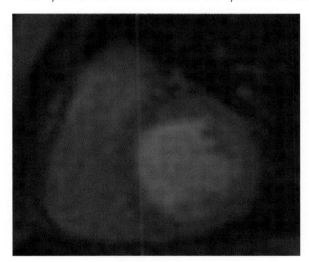

Figure 53-1   First-pass perfusion

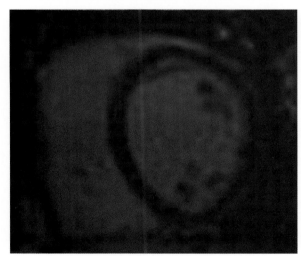

Figure 53-2   Delayed contrast enhancement

Case 53   Stunned/Hibernating Myocardium

Findings

- ► MR:
  - ▪ SSFP: Regional wall hypo-/a-/dyskinesis, reduced systolic thickening, reduced global LV function
  - ▪ FPP: Normal to reduced (only in hibernating) myocardial perfusion
  - ▪ Delayed CE: Normal enhancement through the myocardium
  - ▪ Dobutamine-induced: Enables assessment of contractility reserve to predict LV functional recovery after revascularization

Differential Diagnosis

- ► Normal myocardium
- ► Acute MI with reperfusion
- ► Acute MI without reperfusion
- ► Chronic MI

Teaching Points

- ► Two types
  - ▪ Stunned
    - ◆ Normal myocardial perfusion but decreased function resulting from reperfusion after an ischemic episode
    - ◆ Associated with acute MI
  - ▪ Hibernating
    - ◆ Decreased myocardial perfusion and function resulting from prolonged ischemia or recurrent stunning episodes
    - ◆ Contractility recovers quickly once coronary flow is restored
    - ◆ Associated with high-grade chronic CAD

Management

- ► Coronary revascularization (PCI or CABG) of hibernating myocardium may improve LV function, symptoms, and survival

Further Readings

Camici PG et al. Stunning, hibernation, and assessment of myocardial viability. *Circulation*. 2008;117(1):103–114.

Shan K et al. Role of cardiac magnetic resonance imaging in the assessment of myocardial viability. *Circulation*. 2004;109(11):1328–1334.

History

▶ None

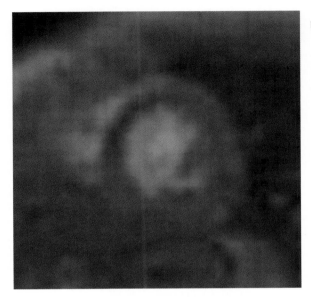

Figure 54-1   First-pass perfusion

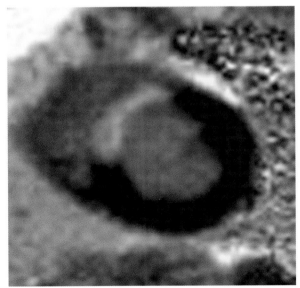

Figure 54-2   Delayed contrast enhancement

Case 54 Transmural Myocardial Infarction

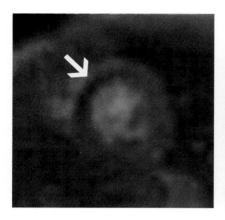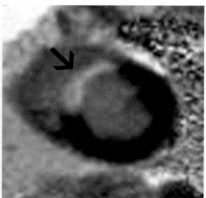

Findings

- MR:
    - T2WI: ± Increased signal intensity (edema) in affected myocardium
    - SSFP: Regional wall hypo-/a-/dyskinesis, reduced systolic thickening
    - FPP: Reduced perfusion of myocardium in the coronary artery distribution (white arrow)
    - Delayed CE: Hyperenhancement of myocardium that extends through the full myocardial thickness (black arrow), ± myocardial thinning

Differential Diagnosis

- Nontransmural MI
- Myocarditis
- Sarcoidosis
- Vasculitis (e.g., Kawasaki disease)
- Nonischemic CM (e.g., dilated CM, restrictive CM)

Teaching Points

- Differentiate acute from chronic transmural MI
    - Acute—normal thickness of the myocardium, myocardial edema
    - Chronic—myocardial thinning, no myocardial edema
- Associated with a poorer prognosis and an increase in complications
- Complications include lethal arrhythmias, mural thrombus, ventricular aneurysm, pseudoaneurysm, or rupture

Management

- Acute: Medical ± endovascular therapy to reperfuse acutely infarcted myocardium
- Chronic: Medical therapy to prevent ventricular remodeling

Further Reading

Sakuma H. Magnetic resonance imaging for ischemic heart disease. *J Magn Reson Imaging.* 2007;26(1):3–13.

History

► None

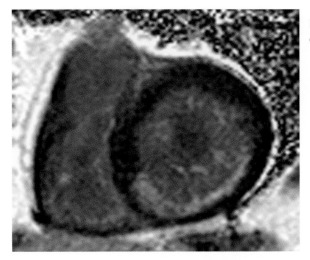

Figure 55-1   Delayed contrast enhancement

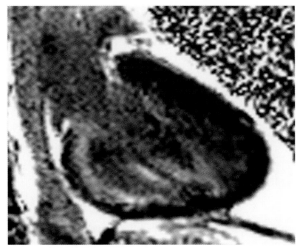

Figure 55-2   Delayed contrast enhancement

Case 55 Nontransmural Myocardial Infarction

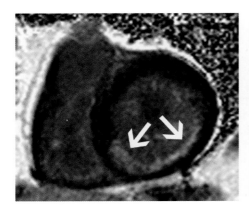 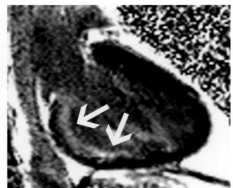

Findings

▸ MR:
  ▪ T2WI: ± Increased signal intensity (edema) in affected myocardium
  ▪ SSFP: Regional wall hypo-/dyskinesis, reduced systolic thickening
  ▪ FPP: Reduced perfusion of myocardium in the coronary artery distribution
  ▪ Delayed CE: Hyperenhancement of myocardium that extends from the subendocardial surface but does not extend through the full thickness of the myocardium (arrows); no myocardial thinning
    ◆ Gold standard for detecting and quantifying nontransmural MI
  ▪ Stress FPP and delayed CE may enable differentiation between MI and stress-induced ischemia (similar to the nuclear medicine stress test)

Differential Diagnosis

▸ Transmural MI
▸ Myocarditis
▸ Sarcoidosis
▸ Vasculitis (e.g., Kawasaki disease)
▸ Nonischemic CM (e.g., dilated CM, restrictive CM)

Teaching Points

▸ Pathologically due to early reperfusion prior to infarction extending transmurally
▸ If ≤50% of the wall thickness in any given segment is infarcted, then functional recovery after revascularization is likely (≥80% likelihood)
▸ Associated with a better prognosis than transmural MI and less frequent complications
▸ Complications: Lethal arrhythmias, mural thrombus, ventricular aneurysm, pseudoaneurysm, or rupture

Management

▸ Early thrombolysis and/or PCI can prevent extension to transmural MI

Further Reading

Vogel-Claussen J et al. Delayed enhancement MR imaging: utility in myocardial assessment. *Radiographics*. 2006;26(3):795–810.

History

▶ A 56-year-old female with a history of MI presents with chest pain

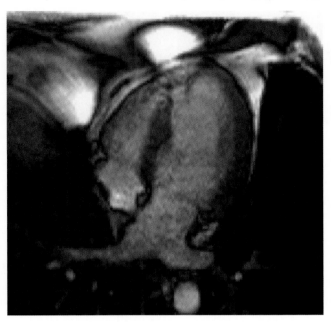

Figure 56-1   Bright blood. Image courtesy of Laura E. Heyneman, MD (Duke University Medical Center, Durham, North Carolina)

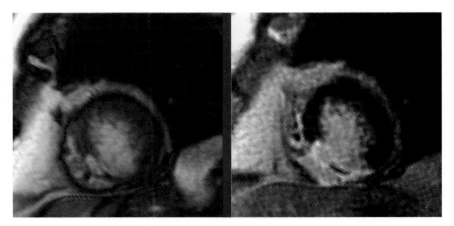

Figure 56-2   Bright blood (left) and delayed contrast enhancement (right) images. Images courtesy of Laura E. Heyneman, MD (Duke University Medical Center, Durham, North Carolina)

Case 56 Ventricular Septal Rupture

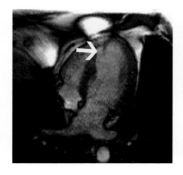 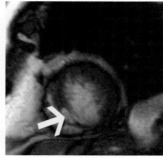 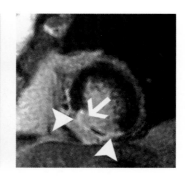

Findings

- ► CXR: Frontal view: RV enlargement, shunt vascularity
- ► CTA/MR: Focal VSD (arrows), regional wall hypo-/akinesis
  - ▪ Delayed CE MR: Transmural hyperenhancement adjacent to the septal defect (arrowheads)

Differential Diagnosis

- ► VSD

Teaching Points

- ► Following acute MI, two types of defects are seen between the LV and RV
  - ▪ Apical septal defect—most common and results from anterior MI; usually a simple, discrete defect
  - ▪ Inferoposterior septal defect—causes higher mortality and results from inferior MI; usually complex, with extensive hemorrhage and serpiginous tracts; occasional tearing of the papillary muscles or ventricular free wall
- ► Earlier reperfusion therapy of acute MI reduces the size of the infarct, decreases the incidence of rupture, and improves the prognosis; however, rupture does occur earlier
- ► Presentation: Recurrent angina, dyspnea, low cardiac output, cardiogenic shock

Management

- ► Medical therapy (intra-aortic balloon pump, afterload reduction, diuretics, inotropic agents) is only for temporary support
- ► Immediate surgical (septal reconstruction) or endovascular (percutaneous closure) therapy to close the septal defect is needed

Further Reading

Birnbaum Y et al. Ventricular septal rupture after acute myocardial infarction. *N Engl J Med.* 2002;347(18):1426–1432.

History

▶ None

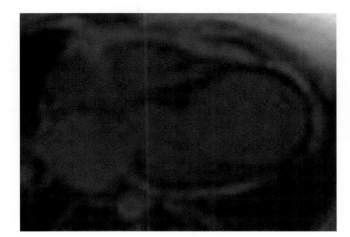

Figure 57-1   Steady-state free precession

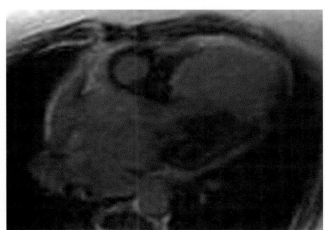

Figure 57-2   Delayed contrast enhancement

Case 57 Left Ventricular Aneurysm

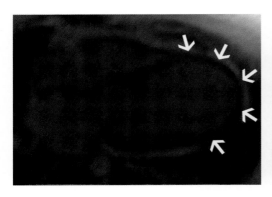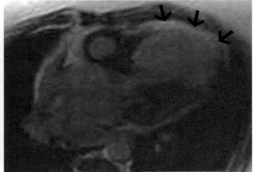

Findings

- ► CXR: Cardiomegaly, bulging myocardial contour, myocardial calcification
- ► CTA: Coronary artery filling defect, reduced wall contractility, myocardial thinning and linear calcifications, dilated LV at the regional wall, neck = maximal diameter of focal dilation
- ► MR:
  - ▪ SSFP: Regional wall dilation and thinning (white arrows) with a-/dyskinesis
  - ▪ FFP: Reduced perfusion of the myocardium in the coronary artery distribution
  - ▪ Delayed CE: Hyperenhancement of transmural myocardium (black arrows)

Differential Diagnosis

- ► LV pseudoaneurysm
- ► Acute MI
- ► Nontransmural MI
- ► Takotsubo cardiomyopathy
- ► Pericardial calcification

Teaching Points

- ► LV dilatation with intact three layers of myocardium due to prior transmural MI; six times higher mortality than in patients without LV aneurysm
- ► Etiology: MI (anterior/apical > inferior-basal/inferolateral)
- ► Associated with mural thrombus
- ► Presentation: Usually asymptomatic
- ► Complications include CHF, lethal ventricular arrhythmias, ventricular rupture, systemic embolization

Management

- ► Medical therapy (e.g., ACE inhibitors, β-blockers) to reduce LV remodeling, control the heart rate, reduce blood pressure, and prevent additional MI
- ► Surgical therapy (e.g., aneurysmectomy, CABG) only in patients with certain complications (e.g., CHF, arrhythmias) but with adequate functional myocardium

Further Reading

Konen E et al. True versus false left ventricular aneurysm: differentiation with MR imaging—initial experience. *Radiology*. 2005;236(1):65–70.

History

▸ None

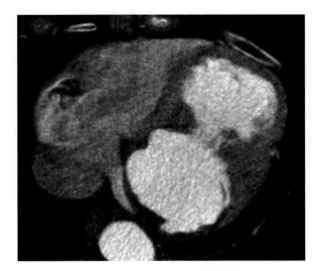

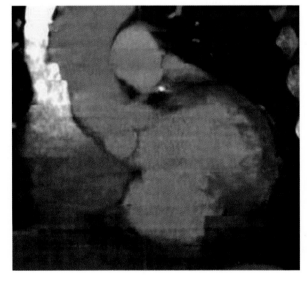

Case 58   Left Ventricular Pseudoaneurysm

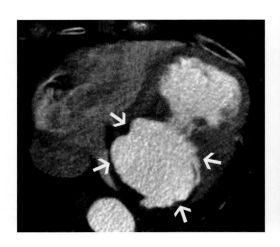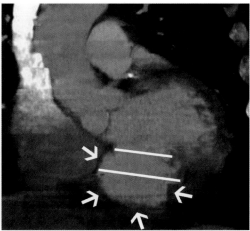

Findings

- ▸ CXR: Rounded or lobulated soft tissue mass in the retrocardiac region (often)
- ▸ CTA: Coronary artery filling defect, focal LV outpouching with a narrow neck (arrows), neck < maximal diameter of the outpouching (lines)
- ▸ MR:
  - ▪ SSFP: Focal LV outpouching, turbulent blood flow in the aneurysm
  - ▪ FFP: Reduced perfusion of myocardium along the border of the orifice
  - ▪ Delayed CE: Hyperenhancement of adjacent epicardium and pericardium along the border of the orifice

Differential Diagnosis

- ▸ LV aneurysm
- ▸ Myocardial tumor

Teaching Points

- ▸ LV outpouching is contained only by the pericardium or scar tissue; both endocardium and myocardium are disrupted
- ▸ The narrow neck is the most useful sign
- ▸ Etiology: MI (inferior > anterior), cardiac surgery, trauma, endocarditis
- ▸ Associated with mural thrombus
- ▸ Presentation: Asymptomatic, angina, dyspnea
- ▸ Complications: LV rupture, CHF, ventricular arrhythmias, syncope, tamponade, sudden death

Management

- ▸ Surgical therapy is the treatment of choice

Further Reading

Frances C et al. Left ventricular pseudoaneurysm. *J Am Coll Cardiol.* 1998;32(3):557–561.

History

▶ A 65-year-old male with a history of chronic CAD

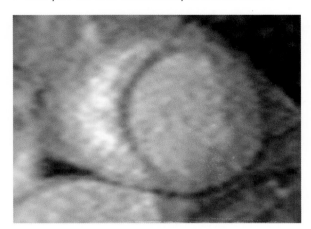

Figure 59-1   First-pass perfusion

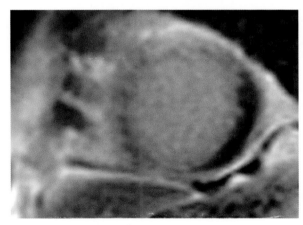

Figure 59-2   Delayed contrast enhancement

Case 59 Ischemic Cardiomyopathy

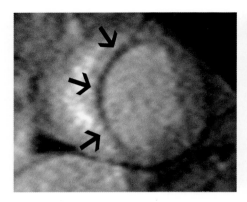 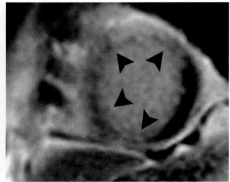

Findings

- ▶ CXR: Globular cardiomegaly, Kerley B lines, cephalization toward the upper lobes, coronary calcification may be visible
- ▶ CTA: Coronary artery filling defect, lower-attenuation myocardium, linear myocardial calcifications, LV dilatation, myocardial thinning, global hypokinesis
- ▶ MR:
  - ▪ SSFP: LV dilatation, global or regional hypokinesis
  - ▪ FPP: Reduced perfusion of the myocardium in the affected coronary artery distribution (arrows)
  - ▪ Delayed CE: Variable transmural and/or nontransmural hyperenhancement of myocardium (arrowheads), myocardial thinning

Differential Diagnosis

- ▶ Dilated CM
- ▶ Chronic myocarditis
- ▶ ARVD (LV involvement)
- ▶ Restrictive CM (e.g., amyloidosis, sarcoidosis)

Teaching Points

- ▶ Caused by significant (multivessel) CAD disease and LV remodeling
- ▶ 50%–60% 5-year survival rate; depends on the ejection fraction (EF), the patient's functional status, and the presence of arrhythmias
- ▶ Presentation: Chest pain, shortness of breath, arrhythmias
- ▶ Complications include LV aneurysm, LV septal rupture, pericardial effusion, valvular regurgitation

Management

- ▶ Medical therapy (e.g., ACE inhibitors, aspirin) to reduce ventricular remodeling and prevent additional MI
- ▶ If there is viable myocardium, coronary revascularization can improve the prognosis
- ▶ Automated implantable cardioverter-defibrillator (AICD) implantation or cardiac transplantation for low EF or arrhythmias

Further Reading

Lipton MJ et al. Imaging of ischemic heart disease. *Eur Radiol.* 2002;12(5):1061–1080.

Part 7

Myocardial Disease—Intrinsic

History

▶ A 64-year-old female with worsening shortness of breath at rest

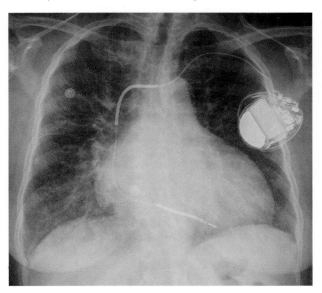

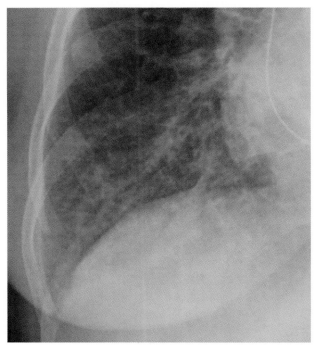

Case 60 Left Heart Failure (CXR)

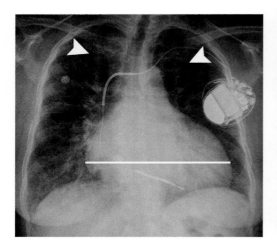 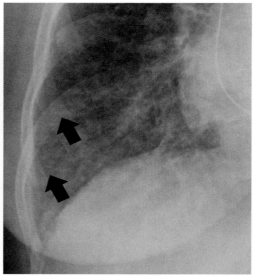

Findings

▶ CXR: Frontal view: Cardiomegaly (line), "cephalization" of the upper lobe vessels (arrowheads), thickening of interlobular septa (arrows), peribronchial thickening or "cuffing", alveolar edema in a "batwing" distribution, ± pleural effusions

Differential Diagnosis

▶ Pneumonia
▶ Acute respiratory distress syndrome
▶ Pericardial effusion
▶ Right heart failure

Teaching Points

▶ Inability of the LV to maintain the stroke volume—preload, myocardial contractility, afterload—resulting in pulmonary edema
▶ Functional assessment is commonly based on the New York Heart Association (NYHA) classification (Classes I to IV)
▶ Although there are currently no standard criteria for diagnosis, the Framingham criteria are commonly used
▶ Etiologies include LV dysfunction (e.g., ischemic CM, nonischemic CM, myocarditis), valvular heart disease (e.g., aortic stenosis, mitral stenosis, mitral regurgitation), HTN
▶ Presentation includes dyspnea on exertion, shortness of breath, cough, orthopnea, paroxysmal nocturnal dyspnea, tachypnea, rales, S3 gallop, tachycardia

Management

▶ *See Case 61: Left Heart Failure (CT)*

Further Readings
See Case 61: Left Heart Failure (CT)

History

▶ A 56-year-old female with new onset of atrial fibrillation and tachypnea

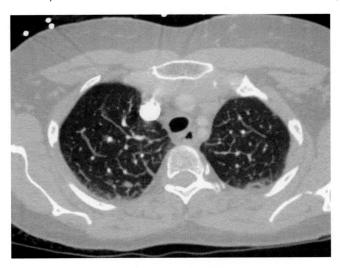

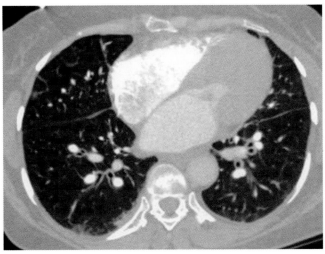

Case 61   Left Heart Failure (CT)

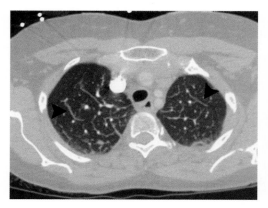 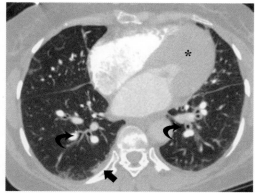

Findings

- High-resolution computed tomography (HRCT): Thickening of interlobular septa (arrowheads), peribronchial thickening or "cuffing" (curved arrows), diffuse ground-glass or alveolar consolidation in a dependent distribution (arrow) ± enlarged mediastinal lymph nodes ± mediastinal fat edema ± pleural effusions
- CTA/MR: Findings of the underlying etiology, such as hypertrophic CM (asterisk), can also assess function (i.e., stroke volume, EF)

Differential Diagnosis

- Pneumonia
- Acute respiratory distress syndrome

Teaching Points

- *See Case 60: Left Heart Failure (CXR)*

Management

- Medical therapy (diuretics, inotropics, ACE inhibitors, β-blockers) to improve symptoms, maintain a euvolemic state, and improve prognosis
- Biventricular pacemakers, AICDs, or left ventricular assisted devices (LVADs) can be used in patients with decreased functional status and a low EF
- Cardiac transplantation for nonresponsive patients

Further Readings

Goodman LR. Congestive heart failure and adult respiratory distress syndrome. New insights using computed tomography. *Radiol Clin North Am.* 1996;34(1):33–46.

Hunt SA et al. 2009 Focused update incorporated into the ACC/AHA 2005 Guidelines for the Diagnosis and Management of Heart Failure in Adults. *J Am Coll Cardiol.* 2009;53(15):e1–e90.

Case 62

History

▶ None

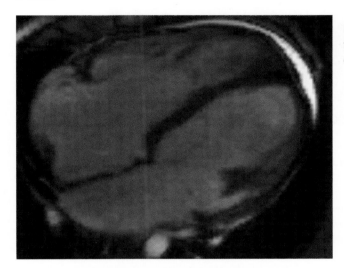

Figure 62-1   Steady-state free precession image in the diastolic phase

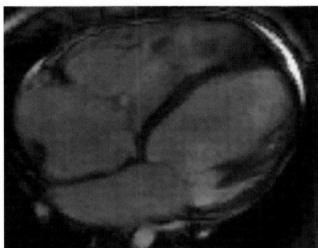

Figure 62-2   Steady-state free precession image in the systolic phase

Case 62 Dilated Cardiomyopathy

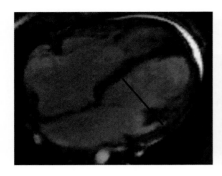 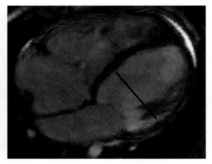

Findings

▶ CXR: Frontal view: Cardiomegaly, "cephalization" of the upper lobe vessels, thickening of interlobular septa, pleural effusions, dilatation of the SVC and the azygos vein
▶ CTA/MR:
  ▪ LV ± RV dilation (lines) and hypokinesis
  ▪ Findings of the underlying etiology (particularly using delayed CE MR to differentiate ischemic from nonischemic dilated CM)
  ▪ Can assess function (i.e., stroke volume, EF)

Differential Diagnosis

▶ Restrictive CM (e.g., amyloidosis, sarcoidosis)
▶ Hypertrophic CM

Teaching Points

▶ LV dilation with systolic dysfunction ± RV dysfunction, low EF (<40%)
▶ Etiology:
  ▪ Primary: Idiopathic (most common worldwide), familial (e.g., Duchenne muscular dystrophy)
  ▪ Secondary: CAD (most common in the United States), valvular heart disease (e.g., aortic stenosis), infection (e.g., coxsackie B virus, Chagas disease), alcohol, cocaine, doxorubicin, amyloidosis, sarcoidosis, thyrotoxicosis, pregnancy, connective tissue disease (e.g., rheumatoid arthritis)
▶ Epidemiology: Median survival is 1.7 years for males and 3.2 years for females; African Americans have a threefold greater risk than whites
▶ Presentation: dyspnea with exertion, orthopnea, paroxysmal nocturnal dyspnea, peripheral edema, arrhythmia, angina
▶ Complication: thromboembolism, sudden death

Management

▶ Treat the underlying etiology
▶ Medical therapy (diuretics, inotropics, ACE inhibitors, β-blockers) to improve LV function and improve the prognosis
▶ Device therapy (e.g., AICD) or cardiac transplantation can be used when medical therapy fails

Further Reading

Jackson E et al. Ischaemic and non-ischaemic cardiomyopathies—cardiac MRI appearances with delayed enhancement. *Clin Radiol.* 2007;62(5):395–403.

History

▶ A 16-year-old male with syncope during exercise

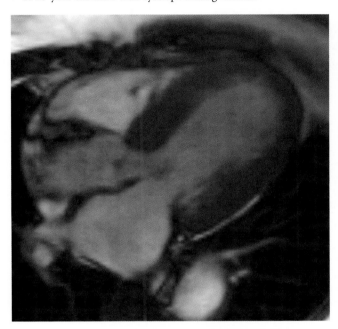

Figure 63-1 Three-chamber steady-state free precession image in the diastolic phase

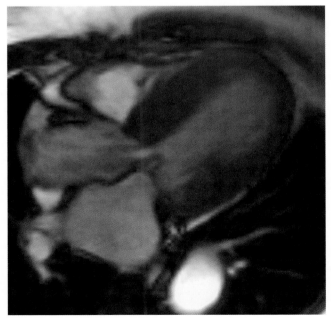

Figure 63-2 Three-chamber steady-state free precession image in the systolic phase

Case 63 Hypertrophic Cardiomyopathy

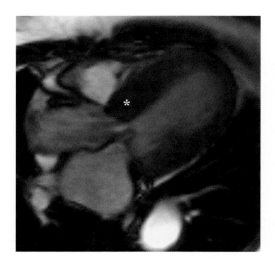

Findings

- ► CXR: Frontal view: Normal to cardiomegaly ± right retrocardiac double density (LA enlargement)
- ► CTA/MR: Asymmetric (asterisk) or symmetric LV myocardial thickening without cavity dilation; involves the basal, middle, apical, or septal aspect of the LV; restrictive diastolic filling of the LV; RV involvement (up to 15%)
    - ▪ SSFP MR: Assess LVOT flow dynamics for obstruction
    - ▪ Delayed CE MR: Focal or diffuse enhancement (fibrosis) within the hypertrophic regions, particularly in the midinterventricular septum

Differential Diagnosis

- ► Aortic stenosis
- ► HTN
- ► Restrictive CM (e.g., amyloidosis, sarcoidosis)

Teaching Points

- ► LV myocardial thickening without an obvious cardiac or systemic etiology
- ► Autosomal dominant, genetic mutation of sarcomeres of the myocardium
- ► Two types
    - ▪ Obstructive:
        - ◆ LVOT obstruction is most commonly due to asymmetric septal hypertrophy, also known as *hypertrophic obstructive cardiomyopathy* (HOCM) or *idiopathic hypertrophic subaortic stenosis* (IHSS)
        - ◆ Dynamic outflow obstruction may occur due to systolic anterior motion (SAM) of the anterior leaflet of the mitral valve
    - ▪ Nonobstructive:
        - ◆ 75% of all hypertrophic CM; apical hypertrophic CM is most common
- ► Presentation: Asymptomatic, exertional dyspnea, atypical chest pain, palpitations, syncope during exercise, atrial fibrillation
- ► Complication: MI, sudden cardiac death in young athletes, likely from ventricular arrhythmias

Management

- ► Medical therapy (β- or calcium channel blockers) to improve diastolic relaxation and reduce the likelihood of arrhythmias
- ► Surgical (septal myomectomy) or endovascular (alcohol septal ablation) therapy when medical therapy fails

Further Reading

Maron BJ. Hypertrophic cardiomyopathy: a systematic review. *JAMA*. 2002;287(10):1308–1320.

History

▶ A 65-year-old male with increasing dyspnea and leg swelling

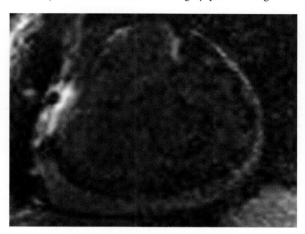

Figure 64-1 Delayed contrast enhancement. Image courtesy of Jean Jeudy, MD (University of Maryland Medical Center, Baltimore, Maryland)

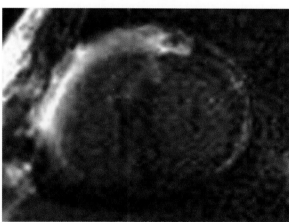

Figure 64-2 Delayed contrast enhancement. Image courtesy of Jean Jeudy, MD (University of Maryland Medical Center, Baltimore, Maryland)

Case 64 Cardiac Amyloidosis

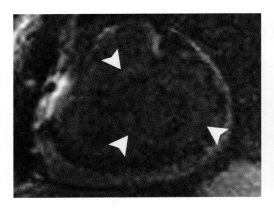 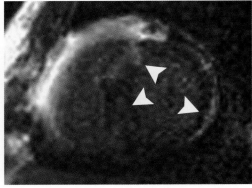

Findings

- ► CTA/MR: Concentric LV ± RV hypertrophy, atrial enlargement, interarterial septal thickening, pericardial and pleural effusions
  - ▪ SSFP MR: Restricted diastolic filling, reduced systolic function (late)
  - ▪ Delayed CE MR: Diffuse heterogeneous enhancement (arrows) of thickened subendocardial myocardium (infiltration, not fibrosis), earlier nulling (inversion time) of affected myocardium in a noncoronary distribution

Differential Diagnosis

- ► Hypertrophic CM
- ► HTN
- ► Other causes of restrictive CM (e.g., cardiac sarcoidosis, hemochromatosis, radiation therapy)
- ► Infiltrative lymphoma

Teaching Points

- ► Most common cause of restrictive CM; also known as *stiff heart syndrome*
- ► Extracellular deposits of various fibrillar protein (e.g., AL, AA), serum amyloid P, and charged glycosaminoglycans, replacing normal tissues
- ► Three major forms of amyloidosis that affect the heart
  - ▪ Primary (amyloid light chain [AL]): Most common; associated with multiple myeloma
  - ▪ Secondary (amyloid associated [AA]): Systemic involvement that can rarely affect the heart
  - ▪ Senile (amyloid Transthyretin [ATTR]): Prevalence increases with age
- ► Amyloid deposits stained with Congo Red dye appear as apple-green birefringence under polarized light
- ► Presentation: Asymptomatic, right heart failure, ascites, peripheral edema, fatigue, dyspnea on exertion, palpitations, conduction abnormalities on the ECG
- ► Diagnosis is confirmed by cardiac biopsy

Management

- ► Diuretics and pacemakers for symptomatic relief
- ► Chemotherapy and/or prednisone have shown some benefits
- ► In certain circumstances, heart (not for AL) or liver transplantation (for ATTR) can be performed

Further Readings

Georgiades CS et al. Amyloidosis: review and CT manifestations. *Radiographics*. 2004;24(2):405–416.
vanden Driesen RI et al. MR findings in cardiac amyloidosis. *AJR Am J Roentgenol.* 2006;186(6):1682–1685.

History

▶ A 40-year-old male presents with syncope and an abnormal ECG

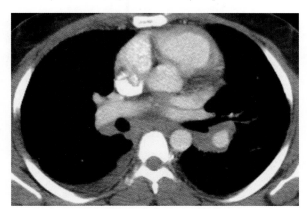

Figure 65-1   Image courtesy of Jean Jeudy, MD (University of Maryland Medical Center, Baltimore, Maryland)

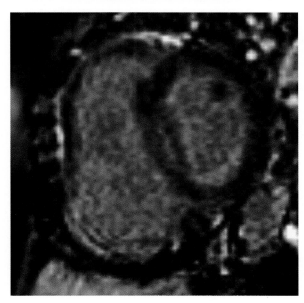

Figure 65-2   Delayed contrast enhancement. Image courtesy of Jean Jeudy, MD (University of Maryland Medical Center, Baltimore, Maryland)

Case 65 Cardiac Sarcoidosis

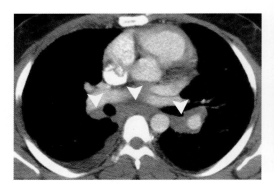
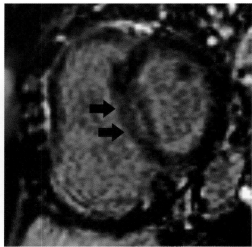

Findings

▶ CXR: Cardiomegaly, hilar lymphadenopathy, prominent interstitial lung markings
▶ CTA/MR: Myocardial thickening (acute inflammation), focal areas of myocardial thinning (chronic, from scarring), hilar lymphadenopathy (arrowheads)
  ▪ T2WI MR: Increased signal intensity (myocardial edema) in the affected and surrounding myocardium (acute), pericardial effusion
  ▪ SSFP MR: Regional or global LV hypo-/dyskinesis
  ▪ FPP/Delayed CE MR: Nodular and patchy subepicardial and midmyocardial hyperenhancement (arrows)

Differential Diagnosis

▶ Hypertrophic CM
▶ Other causes of restrictive CM (e.g., cardiac amyloidosis, hemochromatosis, radiation therapy)
▶ Myocarditis
▶ ARVD

Teaching Points

▶ Noncaseating granulomas involving the peri-/myo-/endocardium
▶ Epidemiology:
  ▪ Young to middle-aged adults; three to four times more likely in African Americans than in whites
  ▪ Cardiac involvement is rarely clinically evident (2%–7%)
  ▪ Serious if symptomatic; the leading cause of death in patients with sarcoidosis (50%–85%)
▶ Presentation: Often asymptomatic, conduction abnormalities and arrhythmias
▶ Complications: Ventricular aneurysms, mitral regurgitation or stenosis, dilated CM, CHF, pericardial tamponade, constrictive pericarditis, sudden death
▶ Diagnosis can be confirmed by cardiac biopsy, although sensitivity is low

Management

▶ Corticosteroids are the mainstay of therapy and may reduce the size of the hyperenhancement on delayed CE MR
▶ Antiarrhythmic therapy and AICD implantation to prevent sudden death

Further Reading

Doughan AR et al. Cardiac sarcoidosis. *Heart*. 2006;92(2):282–288.

History

▶ A 34-year-old male presents after one episode of syncope

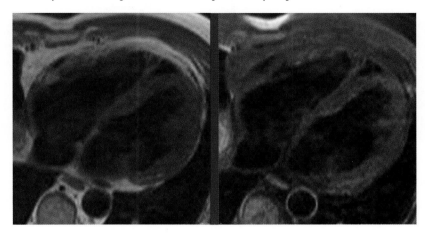

Figure 66-1   T1-weighted images without (left) and with (right) fat saturation. Images courtesy of Jean Jeudy, MD (University of Maryland Medical Center, Baltimore, Maryland)

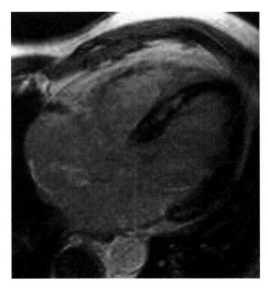

Figure 66-2   Delayed contrast enhancement. Image courtesy of Jean Jeudy, MD (University of Maryland Medical Center, Baltimore, Maryland)

Case 66 Arrhythmogenic Right Ventricular Dysplasia

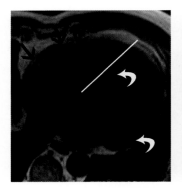 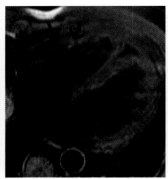 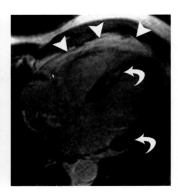

Findings

▶ CTA: Increased RV trabeculation, increased RV intramyocardial fat, scalloping, dilatation of the RV (line) and RVOT, aneurysms of the RV and RVOT
▶ MR:
- T1WI ± FS: RV and RVOT dilatation and/or aneurysm, transmural or islands of fatty infiltration of RV myocardium (arrows) that darkens with fat saturation, diffuse thinning of RV myocardium
- SSFP: global or regional RV systolic and diastolic dysfunction
- Delayed CE: Enhancement of affected myocardium (arrowheads); improves the specificity of MR
- Findings can affect the LV (15%) (curved arrows)

Differential Diagnosis

▶ RV chronic MI
▶ Causes of PA hypertension (e.g., ASD, VSD)
▶ Idiopathic dilated cardiomyopathy
▶ Uhl's anomaly
▶ Normal epicardial fat

Teaching Points

▶ Also known as *arrhythmogenic right ventricular cardiomyopathy* (ARVC)
▶ Pathologically due to fibrofatty or fatty replacement of RV myocardium
▶ Diagnosis based on Task Force criteria (two major, one major and two minor, or four minor)
- Major criteria include RV fatty replacement on pathology or MR (not in original criteria), severe RV dilatation, RV aneurysm
- Minor criteria include mild RV dilatation, regional RV hypokinesis
▶ Epidemiology: Males > females (2.7:1), 30%–50% familial occurrence
▶ Presentation: Syncope, serious ventricular arrhythmias (tachycardia with left bundle branch block [LBBB]), biventricular heart failure, sudden cardiac death

Management

▶ Medical therapy with antiarrhythmic agents is the first treatment option
▶ If medical therapy fails, catheter ablation ± medical therapy is the alternative
▶ Implantable cardioverter-defibrillators (ICDs) are used in patients at high risk of sudden death and those with failed medical therapy
▶ Surgical treatment (e.g., cardiac transplantation) is the last resort

Further Readings

Bomma C et al. Evolving role of multidetector computed tomography in evaluation of arrhythmogenic right ventricular dysplasia/cardiomyopathy. *Am J Cardiol.* 2007;100(1):99–105.
Kayser HW et al. Diagnosis of arrhythmogenic right ventricular dysplasia: a review. *Radiographics.* 2002;22(3):639–648.

History

▶ None

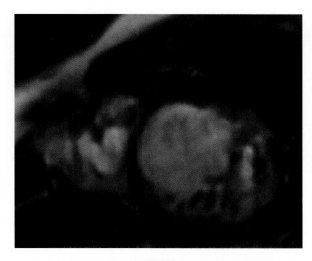

Figure 67-1   Steady-state free precession

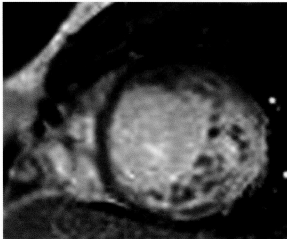

Figure 67-2   Delayed contrast enhancement

Case 67 Left Ventricular Noncompaction

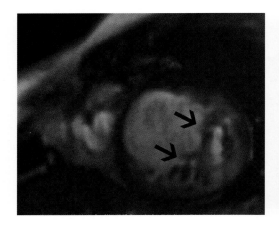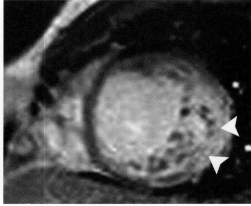

Findings

▶ Location: Apical and mid-LV; can also involve the RV
▶ MR:
  ■ Ratio of noncompacted to compacted myocardium is >2.3:1 (in diastole)
  ■ SSFP: Prominent LV trabeculations with deep intertrabecular recesses (arrows)
  ■ Delayed CE: Trabecular hyperenhancement (arrowheads)

Differential Diagnosis

▶ Dilated CM
▶ Hypertrophic CM
▶ LV thrombus

Teaching Points

▶ Arrest in endomyocardial morphogenesis between 5 and 8 weeks of embryonic life, resulting in failure of compaction of the subendocardial myocardium (from spongy to solid)
▶ Epidemiology: Males > females
▶ Presentation: Ranges from no symptoms to CHF, arrhythmias, and systemic thromboembolic events

Management

▶ Medical (anticoagulants, β-blockers) and surgical (biventricular pacemaker, heart transplantation) treatments are based on the clinical presentation

Further Readings

Dodd JD et al. Quantification of left ventricular noncompaction and trabecular delayed hyperenhancement with cardiac MRI: correlation with clinical severity. *AJR Am J Roentgenol.* 2007;189(4):974–980.
Jassal DS et al. Delayed enhancement cardiac MR imaging in noncompaction of left ventricular myocardium. *J Cardiovasc Magn Reson.* 2006;8(3):489–491.
Petersen SE et al. Left ventricular non-compaction: insights from cardiovascular magnetic resonance imaging. *J Am Coll Cardiol.* 2005;46(1):101–105.
Weiford BC et al. Noncompaction of the ventricular myocardium. *Circulation.* 2004;109(24):2965–2967.

History

▶ A 55-year-old female whose husband recently died

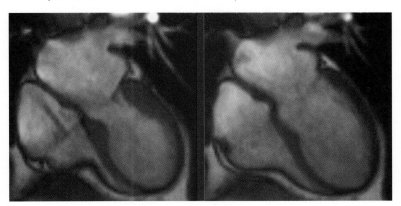

Figure 68-1   Steady-state free precession images in the systolic (left) and diastolic (right) phases. Images courtesy of Jean Jeudy, MD (University of Maryland Medical Center, Baltimore, Maryland)

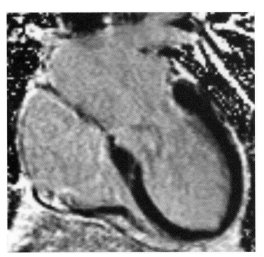

Figure 68-2   Delayed contrast enhancement. Images courtesy of Jean Jeudy, MD (University of Maryland Medical Center, Baltimore, Maryland)

Case 68 Takotsubo Cardiomyopathy

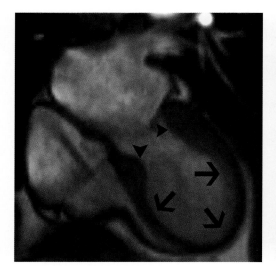 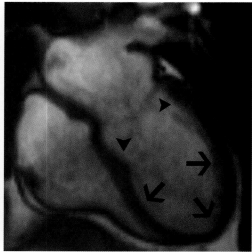

Findings

- ► CTA: No significant (>50%) coronary artery stenosis
- ► MR:
  - SSFP:
    - ◆ Apical ballooning with akinesis or severe hypokinesis of the LV (arrows)
    - ◆ Base of the LV is normal (arrowheads) or hyperkinetic
- ► Delayed CE: Normal

Differential Diagnosis

- ► Acute MI
- ► Acute myocarditis
- ► Dilated CM
- ► Coronary vasospasm

Teaching Points

- ► Also known as *apical ballooning* or *broken heart syndrome*
- ► LV resembles a Japanese pot with a round bottom and a narrow neck used for trapping octopuses
- ► Epidemiology: Frequently occurs in postmenopausal females
- ► Presentation:
  - Mimics acute MI (but negative on coronary angiography); angina, ST-segment elevation, and often elevated cardiac biomarkers
  - Often occurs in settings of acute emotional or physiologic stress

Management

- ► Supportive therapy only; resolves spontaneously within a few weeks

Further Readings

Cummings KW et al. A pattern-based approach to assessment of delayed enhancement in nonischemic cardiomyopathy at MR imaging. *Radiographics.* 2009;29(1):89–103.

Gianni M et al. Apical ballooning syndrome or Takotsubo cardiomyopathy: a systematic review. *Eur Heart J.* 2006;27(13):1523–1529.

History

► A 27-year-old male with recent viral illness presenting with chest pain and ECG changes

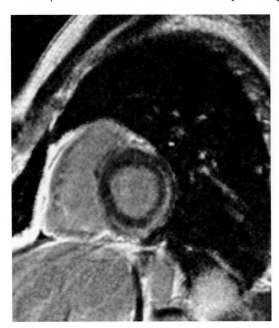

Figure 69-1   Delayed contrast enhancement

Case 69   Myocarditis

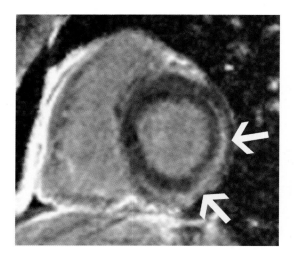

Findings

- ▶ CXR: Cardiomegaly, pulmonary edema
- ▶ CTA: Normal coronary arteries, dilated LV with global systolic dysfunction
- ▶ MR:
  - ▪ T2WI: Increased signal intensity (myocardial edema) in affected walls
  - ▪ SSFP: LV systolic dysfunction
  - ▪ FFP/Delayed CE:
    - ◆ Subepicardial enhancement of affected walls in a noncoronary distribution, frequently involves the lateral wall
    - ◆ Enhancement may not be as intense as in MI

Differential Diagnosis

- ▶ Ischemic CM
- ▶ Dilated CM
- ▶ Restrictive CM (e.g., amyloidosis, sarcoidosis)

Teaching Points

- ▶ Etiology: Viral (most cases), drug toxicities, autoimmune disorders
- ▶ Epidemiology: Postviral infection in an otherwise healthy individual
- ▶ Presentation:
  - ▪ Vague chest pain to fulminant congestive cardiac failure, serious arrhythmias, rarely sudden death
  - ▪ Leukocytosis, elevated erythrocyte sedimentation rate and cardiac biomarkers

Management

- ▶ Majority of patients recover fully with supportive therapy, although one-third of patients will develop dilated CM requiring cardiac transplantation

Further Readings

Cummings KW et al. A pattern-based approach to assessment of delayed enhancement in nonischemic cardiomyopa-thy at MR imaging. *Radiographics.* 2009;29(1):89–103.

Vogel-Claussen J et al. Delayed enhancement MR imaging: utility in myocardial assessment. *Radiographics.* 2006;26(3):795–810.

History

▶ A 71-year-old male after a high-velocity motor vehicle collision

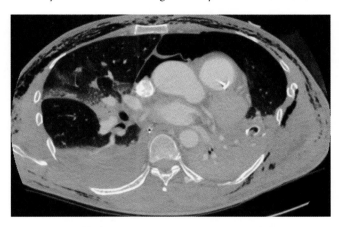

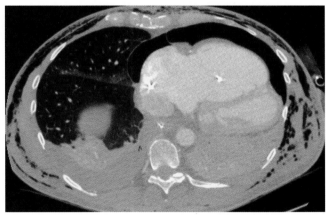

Case 70   Cardiac Herniation

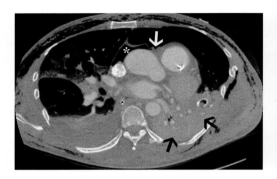
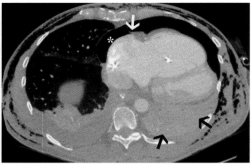

Findings

- CXR:
    - Initial CXR may appear normal or show nonspecific abnormalities
    - Unusual cardiac silhouette, change in cardiac position after chest tube placement
- CT:
    - Cardiac displacement to the side of the herniation (left > right) with ipsilateral atelectasis (black arrows), pneumomediastinum, pneumopericardium (asterisks); these findings can often be seen on CXR
    - Cardiac axis deviation, focal pericardial discontinuity (white arrows)
    - Waist around the compressed portion of the heart herniating through the pericardial defect (collar sign)
    - Air outlining the empty pleuropericardium as a result of the dislocation of the heart into the hemithorax (empty pericardial sac sign)
    - Signs of cardiac tamponade, including a deformed ventricular contour, a dilated IVC, reflux of contrast into the IVC, periportal lymphedema, pericholecystic fluid, ascites

Differential Diagnosis

- LV aneurysm
- RV hypertrophy
- Pericardial mass (e.g., pericardial cyst, pericardial hematoma)
- Partially/completely absent pericardium

Teaching Points

- Etiology:
    - High-energy blunt trauma to the chest creating a pericardial defect
    - In turn, the heart herniates through the defect, causing constriction of the cardiac chambers, coronary vessels, and/or great vessels
- Epidemiology: Rare (<1% of all traumas); most patients die prior to hospitalization; mortality up to 43% in hospitalized patients
- Presentation:
    - Sudden hemodynamic instability such as fluctuating blood pressures or tachycardia, cardiogenic shock, dilated internal jugular vein
    - Small defects are more likely than large defects to be symptomatic

Management

- Thoracotomy for reduction of the cardiac herniation

Further Readings

Nassiri N et al. Imaging of cardiac herniation in traumatic pericardial rupture. *J Thorac Imaging*. 2009;24(1):69–72.
Wielenberg AJ et al. Cardiac herniation due to blunt trauma: early diagnosis facilitated by CT. *AJR Am J Roentgenol*. 2006;187(2):W239–W240.

Part 8

Myocardial Disease—Tumors and Tumor-like Conditions

History

▶ A 40-year-old male with a history of atrial fibrillation

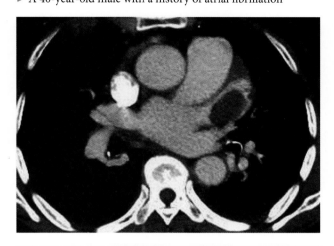

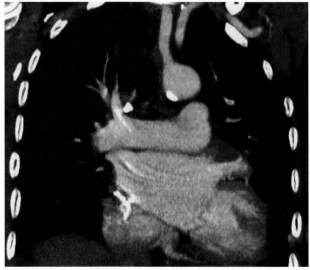

Case 71 Left Atrial Thrombus

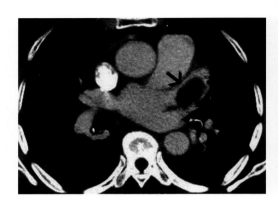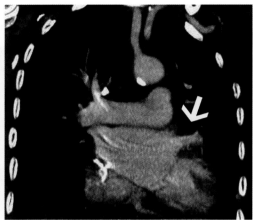

Findings

- ► Location: Left atrial appendage (most common), body of the left atrium
- ► CTA: Persistent homogeneous low-density filling defect without enhancement (arrows)
- ► MR:
  - ▪ T1WI, T2WI: Variable signal intensity, depending on the age of the thrombus
  - ▪ FFP, Delayed CE: Generally, thrombi do not enhance after gadolinium contrast administration, although some may show peripheral enhancement

Differential Diagnosis

- ► Technical artifacts
- ► Cardiac tumors (e.g., myxoma, metastasis)

Teaching Points

- ► Mixing artifacts can be eliminated by acquiring delayed CT images
- ► Etiology: Atrial fibrillation, mitral valve disease, ASD closure device
- ► Presentation: Asymptomatic, cerebral stroke or transient ischemic attack, other embolic events (e.g., superior mesenteric artery occlusion)

Management

- ► Anticoagulation can reduce the risk of an embolic event and dissolve the thrombus
- ► Surgical (e.g., the Cox maze procedure) or endovascular (e.g., radiofrequency ablation) therapy to treat atrial fibrillation
- ► Surgical or endovascular obliteration of the left atrial appendage

Further Readings

Scheffel H et al. Atrial myxomas and thrombi: comparison of imaging features on CT. *AJR Am J Roentgenol.* 2009;192(3):639–645.
Sparrow PJ et al. MR imaging of cardiac tumors. *Radiographics.* 2005;25(5):1255–1276.

History

▶ A 67-year-old male with prior inferior MI

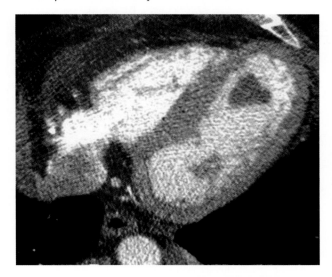

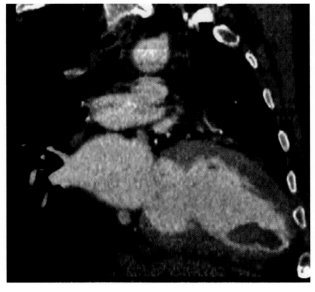

Case 72 Left Ventricular Thrombus

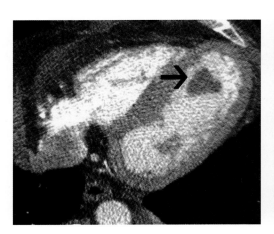 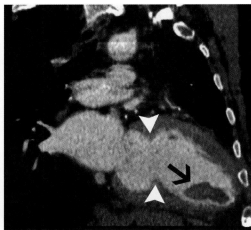

Findings

▶ CTA: Persistent homogeneous low-density filling defect without enhancement (arrows), ± associated findings of MI, such as LV aneurysm (arrowheads)
▶ MR:
- T1WI, T2WI: Variable signal intensity, depending on the age of the thrombus
- SSFP: May exhibit mobility
- FFP, Delayed CE: Generally, thrombi do not enhance after gadolinium contrast administration

Differential Diagnosis

▶ Papillary muscles
▶ Technical artifacts
▶ Cardiac tumors (e.g., myxoma, metastasis)

Teaching Points

▶ Papillary muscle moves with the myocardium, while thrombus does not
▶ Etiology: Poor LV wall motion, such as in patients with prior MI, ventricular aneurysm, cardiomyopathy
▶ Presentation: Asymptomatic, cerebral stroke or transient ischemic attack, other embolic events (e.g., superior mesenteric artery occlusion)

Management

▶ Anticoagulation can potentially reduce the risk of an embolic event and dissolve the thrombus

Further Reading

Weinsaft JW et al. Detection of left ventricular thrombus by delayed-enhancement cardiovascular magnetic resonance prevalence and markers in patients with systolic dysfunction. *J Am Coll Cardiol.* 2008;52(2):148–157.

History

▸ None

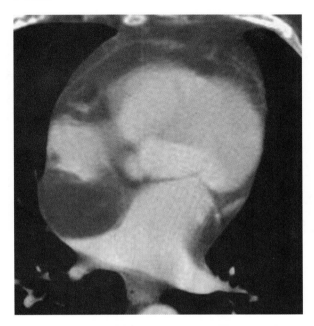

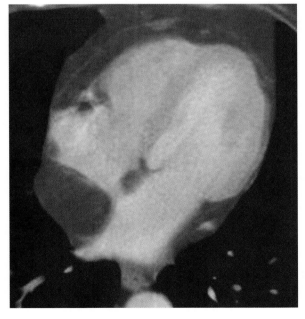

Case 73 Lipomatous Hypertrophy of Interatrial Septum

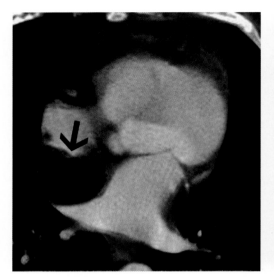 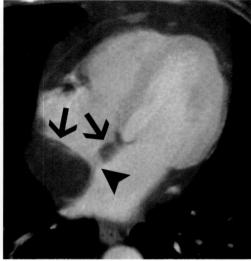

Findings

- ► CTA: Mass-like fat accumulation within the interatrial septum (arrows), sparing the fossa ovalis (arrowhead), characteristically dumbbell-shaped
- ► MR: T1WI: Hyperintense lesion; signal dropout with fat saturation

Differential Diagnosis

- ► Cardiac tumors (e.g., myxoma, fibroma, lipoma, liposarcoma)
- ► Atrial thrombus
- ► Cardiac metastases
- ► Teratoma
- ► MI

Teaching Points

- ► Caused by excessive deposition of fat within the interatrial septum
- ► Unencapsulated compared to other fat-containing masses
- ► Epidemiology: More common in advanced age and in obese patients
- ► Presentation: Usually asymptomatic, rarely cause obstruction of the right tricuspid valve, exertional dyspnea, syncope, supraventricular arrhythmias, and sudden cardiac death

Management

- ► None; usually a benign incidental finding
- ► If it is clinically significant, surgical resection can be performed

Further Readings

Gaerte SC et al. Fat-containing lesions of the chest. *Radiographics*. 2002;22 Spec No:S61–S78.
Meaney JF et al. CT appearance of lipomatous hypertrophy of the interatrial septum. *AJR Am J Roentgenol*. 1997;168(4):1081–1084.

History

▶ A 40-year-old female present with orthopnea

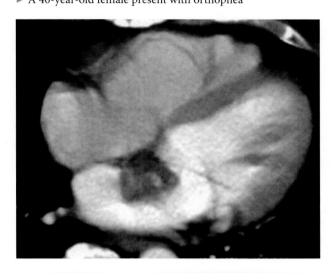

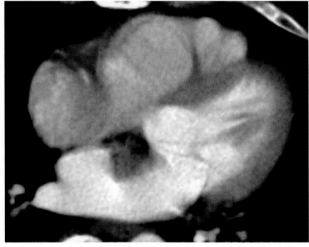

Case 74 Atrial Myxoma

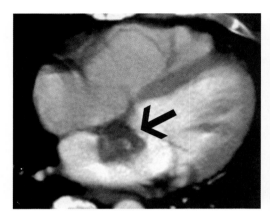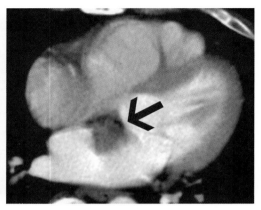

Findings

- ► Location: LA (60%), RA, rarely venticles
- ► CXR: Cardiomegaly, pulmonary edema, intracardiac calcifications
- ► CTA: Low-density, heterogeneous, ovoid mass with a lobular contour in the left atrium extending from the atrial septum (arrows), usually a stalk from the fossa ovalis; may have calcification or cystic components; generally does not enhance
- ► MR:
  - ▪ T1WI: Heterogeneous hypointense mass
  - ▪ T2WI: Heterogeneous hyperintense mass
  - ▪ SSFP: Characteristic mobility of the mass; may prolapse across the mitral or tricuspid valve
  - ▪ T1+Gad: Heterogeneous enhancement of the mass

Differential Diagnosis

- ► Atrial thrombus
- ► Other cardiac tumors (e.g., lipoma, metastasis, papillary fibroelastoma)

Teaching Points

- ► Most common primary tumor of the heart
- ► Usually sporadic; rarely associated with the Carney complex—myxomas, hyperpigmented skin lesions, and extracardiac tumors (e.g., pituitary adenomas, breast fibroadenomas, melanotic schwannomas)
- ► Epidemiology: Females (60%)
- ► Presentation: Obstructive symptoms resulting from mitral or, less commonly, tricuspid stenosis; nonspecific symptoms include fatigue, weight loss, fever
- ► Complications: Cerebral stroke, other embolic events

Management

- ► Surgical resection (median sternotomy) of the mass

Further Reading

Grebenc ML et al. Cardiac myxoma: imaging features in 83 patients. *Radiographics*. 2002;22(3):673–689.

History

▸ A 1-month-old male with a history of seizures and cardiac murmurs

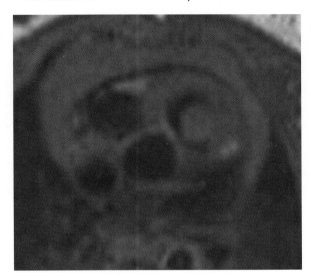

Figure 75-1   T1-weighted

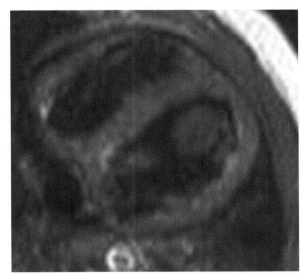

Figure 75-2   T1-weighted

Case 75 Cardiac Rhabdomyoma

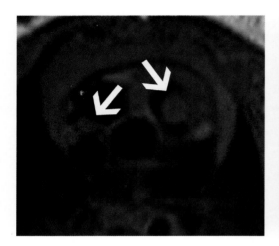 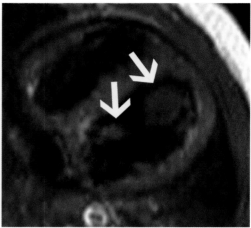

Findings

- ► CTA: Smooth, broad-based, hypodense single or multiple masses arising in the myocardium, most commonly from the ventricles
- ► MR:
  - ▪ T1WI: Solid, homogeneous mass, hypo- to isointense to the myocardium (arrows)
  - ▪ T2WI: Slightly hyperintense mass
  - ▪ FFP: No to minimal enhancement of the mass
  - ▪ Delayed CE: Hyperenhancement of the mass

Differential Diagnosis

- ► Ventricular thrombus
- ► Other cardiac tumors (e.g., fibroma, metastasis)

Teaching Points

- ► Benign myocardial hamartomas
- ► MR is used for surgical planning; usually diagnosed by prenatal ultrasound (US)
- ► Associated with tuberous sclerosis (50%–65%), especially with multiple masses
- ► Epidemiology: ≤90% of cardiac tumors in children, usually <1 year old
- ► Presentation: Most are asymptomatic; arrhythmias, murmurs, heart failure

Management

- ► Often regresses spontaneously
- ► Surgical resection is considered in life-threatening cases

Further Readings

O'Donnell DH et al. Cardiac tumors: optimal cardiac MR sequences and spectrum of imaging appearances. *AJR Am J Roentgenol.* 2009;193(2):377–387.

Umeoka S et al. Pictorial review of tuberous sclerosis in various organs. *Radiographics.* 2008;28(7):e32.

History

▶ A 40-year-old male with dyspnea

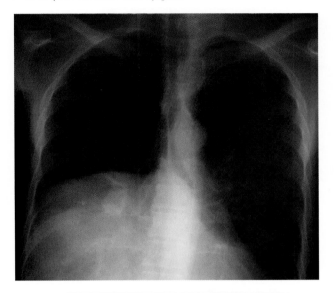

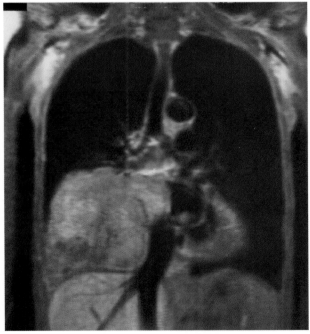

Case 76 Cardiac Angiosarcoma

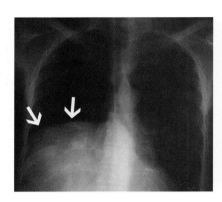 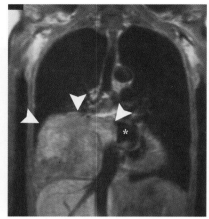

Findings

▶ Two morphologic types:
- Large, well-defined mass (80%) arising from the free wall of the RA with necrosis, hemorrhage, and myocardial, pericardial, and mediastinal invasion
- Diffusely infiltrating mass extending along the pericardium

▶ CXR: Right-sided cardiomegaly, hilar adenopathy, pulmonary edema, pleural effusion, local invasion (arrows) and metastases

▶ CTA: Large, irregular, lobulated, low-attenuation mass, pericardial thickening or (hemorrhagic) effusion, heterogeneous enhancement

▶ MR:
- T1WI, T2WI: Mass (arrowheads) with hyperintense signal interspersed within areas of intermediate signal ("cauliflower" appearance) arising from the RA (asterisk)
- T1+Gad: Heterogeneous enhancement; rarely, linear enhancement extends from the epicardium to the pericardium ("sunray" appearance)

Differential Diagnosis

▶ Other malignant cardiac tumors (e.g., metastasis, lymphoma)

Teaching Points

▶ Most common cardiac sarcomas (37%), the most common primary malignant cardiac tumors
▶ All other types of sarcoma are found more commonly in the LA
▶ Rapid growth, invasion of adjacent structures, and metastasis; survival range is 3 months to 1 year
▶ Epidemiology: Males > females (2:1), mainly affects middle-aged adults
▶ Presentation: Right-sided heart failure or tamponade; nonspecific symptoms of fever and weight loss
▶ Complications: Arrhythmia, myocardial rupture, tamponade (hemopericardium), pulmonary metastases

Management

▶ Surgical resection for palliation and survival benefit, although recurrence and metastases usually occur within <1 year

Further Readings

Araoz PA et al. CT and MR imaging of primary cardiac malignancies. *Radiographics*. 1999;19(6):1421–1434.
O'Donnell DH et al. Cardiac tumors: optimal cardiac MR sequences and spectrum of imaging appearances. *AJR Am J Roentgenol*. 2009;193(2):377–387.

History

▶ None

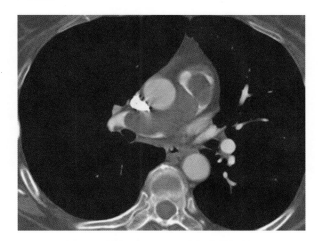

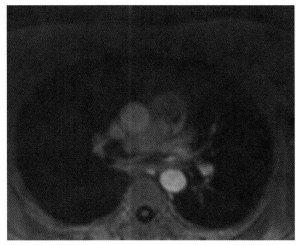

Figure 77-2   Postcontrast T1-weighted image with fat saturation

Case 77 Pulmonary Artery Sarcoma

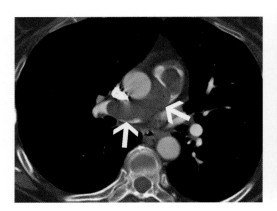 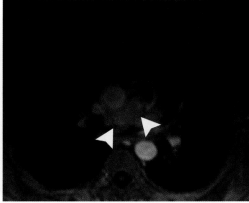

Findings

- ► CXR: Frontal view: Hilar/PA enlargement, pulmonary nodules, enlargement of the cardiac/pericardial contour, decreased pulmonary vascularity
- ► CTA/MR:
  - ▪ Unilateral intraluminal filling defect in the main or proximal PA (arrows) with some enhancement (arrowheads); the filling defect may span the entire luminal diameter
  - ▪ Enlargement or lobularity of the PA
  - ▪ Local extension and metastases

Differential Diagnosis

- ► Pulmonary embolism
- ► Hilar adenopathy
- ► Metastases
- ► Mediastinal fibrosis

Teaching Points

- ► Malignancy of the wall of the PA
- ► Enhancement allows differentiation from pulmonary embolism
- ► Undifferentiated sarcoma or leiomyosarcoma are the most common types
- ► Associated with a very poor prognosis
- ► Presentation: Dyspnea, chest/back pain, cough, hemoptysis, systolic murmur, RV hypertrophy
- ► Complications: Pulmonary infarcts from thrombi or embolization of the tumor

Management

- ► Surgical resection
- ► No thrombolytic therapy—may result in life-threatening hemorrhage

Further Readings

Cox JE et al. Pulmonary artery sarcomas: a review of clinical and radiologic features. *J Comput Assist Tomogr.* 1997;21(5):750–755.

Remy-Jardin M et al. Spiral CT angiography of the pulmonary circulation. *Radiology.* 1999;212(3): 615–636.

History

▶ A 60-year-old male with dyspnea and facial and arm swelling

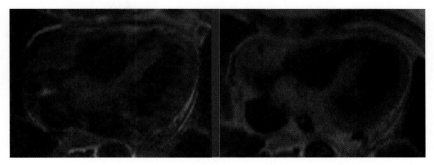

Figure 78-1 Precontrast (left) and postcontrast (right) T1-weighted images

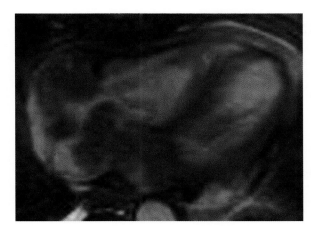

Figure 78-2 Bright blood

Case 78 Cardiac Lymphoma

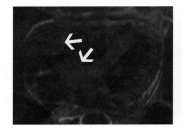 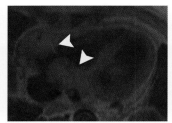 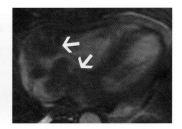

Findings

- ► Large, lobulated mass or diffuse infiltration of myocardium
- ► Location: RA (most common in primary lymphoma), although it often involves other chamber(s) (75%) and the pericardium; the pericardium is frequently involved in secondary lymphoma
- ► CXR: Cardiomegaly, pericardial effusion, signs of heart failure
- ► CTA/MR: Hypo- or isodense/intense mass (arrows), heterogeneous enhancement (arrowheads), pericardial effusion, encasement of the coronary artery, extracardiac involvement (secondary lymphoma)

Differential Diagnosis

- ► Other cardiac tumors (e.g., myxoma, angiosarcoma, metastasis)
- ► Hypertrophic CM

Teaching Points

- ► Etiology:
  - ▪ Primary: Rarely, non-Hodgkin's lymphoma involving the heart or pericardium; most frequently seen in immunocompromised patients (e.g., HIV/AIDS, transplant patients)
  - ▪ Secondary: More common; 16%–28% of patients with systemic lymphoma, second most common metastastic disease to the heart
- ► Presentation: Dyspnea, arrhythmia, SVC obstruction, rapidly worsening heart failure, chest pain; frequently asymptomatic in secondary lymphoma

Management

- ► Early medical treatment with chemotherapy improves the prognosis

Further Readings

Ceresoli GL et al. Primary cardiac lymphoma in immunocompetent patients: diagnostic and therapeutic management. *Cancer.* 1997;80(8):1497–1506.

Grebenc ML et al. Primary cardiac and pericardial neoplasms: radiologic–pathologic correlation. *Radiographics.* 2000;20(4):1073–1103.

History

▶ A 52-year-old male with dyspnea and peripheral edema

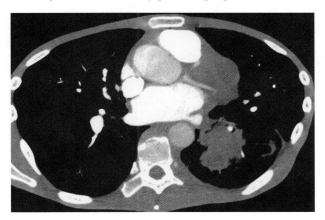

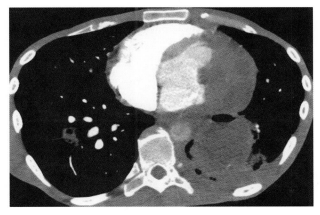

Case 79 Cardiac Metastases

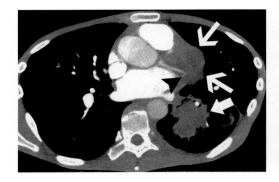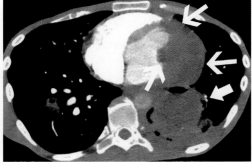

Findings

▶ Location: Epicardium and pericardium, followed by myocardium
▶ CTA: Lobular mass, pericardial (hemorrhagic or serosanguineous) effusion or nodularity (arrows), local invasion, vascular involvement (arrowhead), extracardiac involvement (block arrows)
▶ MR:
  ▪ T1WI: Hypointense mass, except for melanoma (hyperintense on T1WI)
  ▪ T2WI: Hyperintense mass
  ▪ T1+Gad: Heterogeneous enhancement

Differential Diagnosis

▶ Pericarditis (e.g., radiation-induced, drug-induced, idiopathic)
▶ Other cardiac tumors (e.g., fibroma, angiosarcoma)
▶ Thrombus

Teaching Points

▶ Secondary cardiac malignancy from contiguous spread (most common), retrograde lymphatic drainage, hematogenous seeding, or transvenous extension
▶ Epidemiology:
  ▪ 20–40 times more common than primary cardiac tumors
  ▪ Occurs in 10%–12% of all patients with known malignancies
▶ Bronchogenic carcinoma (most common), lymphoma, leukemia, breast cancer, esophageal cancer, melanoma, renal cell carcinoma, sarcoma
▶ Presentation: Most commonly asymptomatic; dyspnea, cough, chest pain, or peripheral edema, arrhythmia
▶ Complications: Pericardial tamponade, CHF, coronary artery invasion, or SA node invasion

Management

▶ If the diagnosis of pericardial effusion is unclear, pericardiocentesis and/or pericardioscopy can be performed
▶ Palliative treatment using chemotherapy or radiation therapy

Further Reading

Chiles C et al. Metastatic involvement of the heart and pericardium: CT and MR imaging. *Radiographics.* 2001;21(2):439–449.

Part 9

Cardiac Valvular Disease

History

▶ None

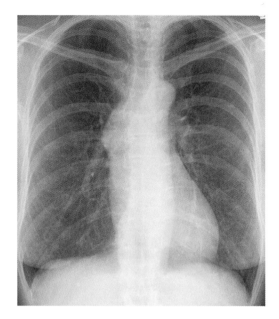

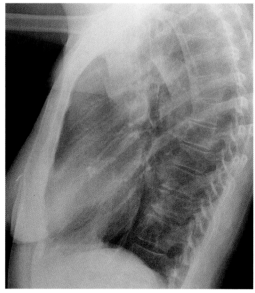

Case 80 Aortic Valve Stenosis (CXR)

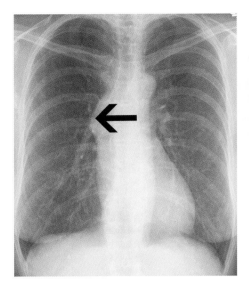 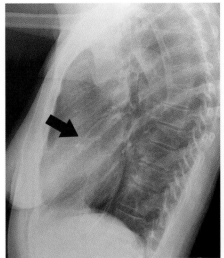

Findings

▶ CXR:
  ▪ Frontal view: Cardiomegaly, rounding of the LV free wall, elevated LV apex, poststenotic dilatation of the ascending aorta (arrow)
  ▪ Lateral view: Calcification of the aortic valve (block arrow)

Differential Diagnosis

▶ Ascending aortic aneurysm
▶ Ascending aortic dissection
▶ Right hilar adenopathy (for the ascending aortic contour)

Teaching Points

▶ Gradual narrowing of the aortic valve area resulting in obstruction of flow from the LV to the ascending aorta during systole
▶ Severity of stenosis is based on aortic jet velocity, mean pressure gradient, and valve area
▶ Etiology:
  ▪ Congenital: Bicuspid (most common in younger patients)
  ▪ Acquired: Age-related degeneration (most common in elderly patients), rheumatic heart disease (often associated with mitral valve disease)
▶ Presentation:
  ▪ Usually asymptomatic until late
  ▪ Angina, syncope, dyspnea
  ▪ Systolic heart murmur, carotid pulsus parvus et tardus
▶ Complications: CHF, sudden death

Management

▶ Aortic valve replacement improves the prognosis, with 85% 10-year survival

Further Reading
See Case 81: Aortic Valve Stenosis (CT).

History

▶ None

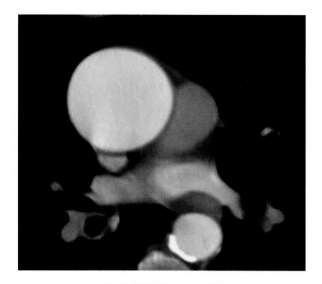

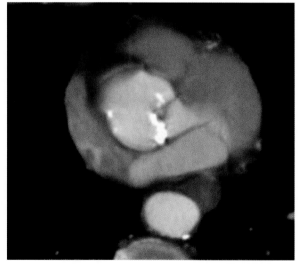

Case 81 Aortic Valve Stenosis (CT)

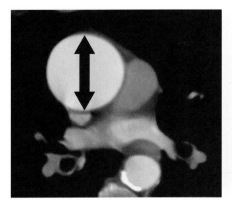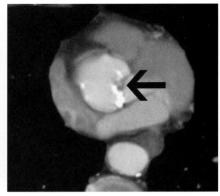

Findings

- CT:
  - NECT: Quantification of aortic valve calcification is associated with aortic stenosis severity
  - CTA:
    - Thickening and calcification of the aortic valve cusps (arrow), leaflet deformity and doming
    - Reduction of the aortic valve area on planimetry
    - Compensatory changes—poststenotic dilatation of the ascending aorta (double arrow), concentric LV hypertrophy
    - Cine: Decreased excursion of valve cusps during the systolic phase
- MR:
  - Thickening of aortic valve cusps, compensatory changes
  - SSFP: Systolic flow void across the stenosis, decreased excursion of valve cusps during the systolic phase
  - Phase contrast: Increased flow velocity and flow gradient across the stenosis

Differential Diagnosis

- Hypertrophic CM
- Ascending aortic aneurysm (primary causes)

Teaching Points

- *See Case 80: Aortic Valve Stenosis (CXR)*

Management

- *See Case 80: Aortic Valve Stenosis (CXR)*

Further Readings

Manghat NE et al. Imaging the heart valves using ECG-gated 64-detector row cardiac CT. *Br J Radiol.* 2008;81(964):275–290.

Pouleur AC et al. Aortic valve area assessment: multidetector CT compared with cine MR imaging and transthoracic and transesophageal echocardiography. *Radiology.* 2007;244(3):745–754.

Vogel-Claussen J et al. Cardiac valve assessment with MR imaging and 64-section multi-detector row CT. *Radiographics.* 2006;26(6):1769–1784.

Willmann JK et al. Electrocardiographically gated multi-detector row CT for assessment of valvular morphology and calcification in aortic stenosis. *Radiology.* 2002;225(1):120–128.

History

▶ A 33-year-old asymptomatic male with wide pulse pressure and a holodiastolic murmur

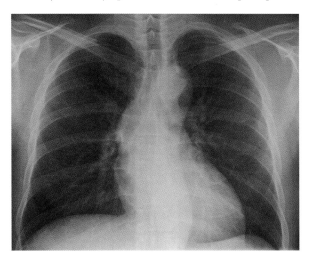

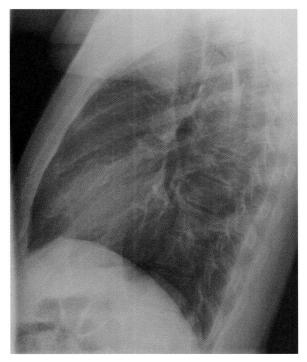

Case 82 Aortic Regurgitation (CXR)

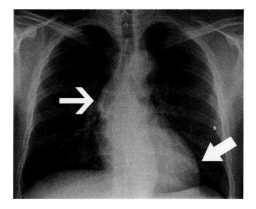

Findings

- ▶ CXR: Frontal view:
  - ▪ Acute: Normal heart size, pulmonary edema
  - ▪ Chronic: LV enlargement (laterally and inferiorly) (block arrow—*subtle finding*), dilatation of the ascending aorta (arrow)

Differential Diagnosis

- ▶ Dilated CM
- ▶ Left heart failure

Teaching Points

- ▶ Poor coaptation of the aortic valve cusps allowing leakage of blood from the aorta to the LV during diastole
- ▶ Volume overload causing LV and aortic dilatation
- ▶ Etiology:
  - ▪ Intrinsic to the valve: Age-related degeneration (most common), bicuspid valve, rheumatic heart disease, bacterial endocarditis
  - ▪ Aortic root: Marfan syndrome (most common in patients <40 years old), idiopathic dilatation of the aortic annulus, systemic HTN, syphilitic aortitis, aortic aneurysm, aortic dissection, trauma
- ▶ Presentation:
  - ▪ Usually asymptomatic until late; chest or abdominal pain, wide pulse pressure, high-pitched holodiastolic decrescendo heart murmur
- ▶ Complication: LV dysfunction and failure

Management

- ▶ Medical therapy (digoxin, diuretics, vasodilator) to eliminate symptoms and possibly delay surgery
- ▶ Aortic valve replacement should be performed in symptomatic patients or in asymptomatic patients with LV dysfunction
- ▶ In certain cases, the treatment should be targeted to the underlying etiology (e.g., long-term antibiotics for endocarditis)

Further Reading

See Case 83: Aortic Regurgitation (MR).

History

▶ None

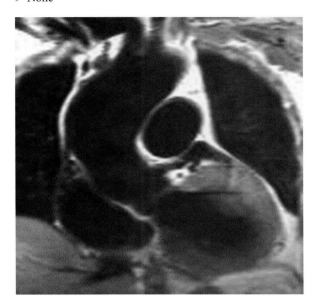

Figure 83-1   T1-weighted

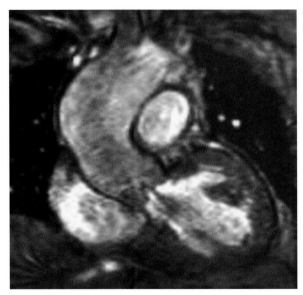

Figure 83-2   Steady-state free precession

Case 83 Aortic Regurgitation (MR)

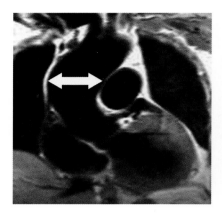 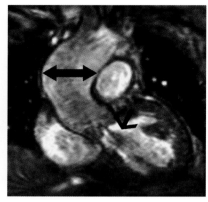

Findings

▶ CTA:
  - Malcoaptation of aortic valve cusps during mid- to end-diastole
  - Pulmonary edema (acute), concentric or eccentric LV hypertrophy to LV dilatation (chronic)
  - Findings of the underlying etiology (e.g., thickening and calcification of aortic valve cusps, effacement of the sinotubular junction, aortic intimal flap)
  - Cine: Increased EF

▶ MR:
  - Malcoaptation of aortic valve cusps, concentric or eccentric LV hypertrophy to LV dilatation, findings of the underlying etiology such as ascending aortic dilatation (double arrow)
  - SSFP MR: Retrograde flow void in diastole across the incompletely coapted aortic valves (arrow)
  - Phase-contrast MR:
    - Increased EF
    - Assess the volume of regurgitation—a flow velocity map is generated on which antegrade and retrograde blood flows appear white and black, respectively, while stationary tissue appears gray; retrograde flow can then be identified and quantified

Differential Diagnosis

▶ Dilated CM
▶ Left heart failure

Teaching Points

▶ *See Case: Aortic Regurgitation (CXR)*

Management:

▶ *See Case 82: Aortic Regurgitation (CXR)*

Further Readings

Didier D et al. Detection and quantification of valvular heart disease with dynamic cardiac MR imaging. *Radiographics*. 2000;20(5):1279–1299.
Feuchtner GM et al. 64-MDCT for diagnosis of aortic regurgitation in patients referred to CT coronary angiography. *AJR Am J Roentgenol*. 2008;191(1):W1–W7.

History

▶ None

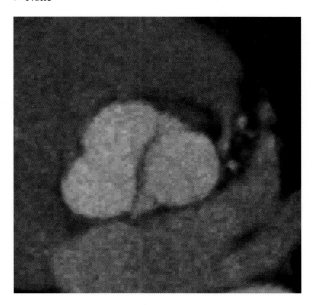

Case 84 Bicuspid Aortic Valve

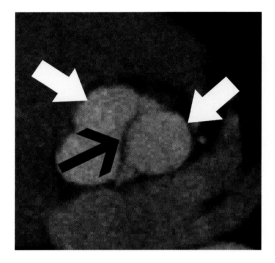

Findings

- ► CXR: Frontal view: Cardiomegaly, poststenotic dilatation of the ascending aorta
- ► CTA/MR: Two separate cusps of unequal size (white arrows) ± a single fused commissure, "fish mouth" appearance (short axis) and "doming" (long axis) of the aortic valve during systole, ± associated findings or complications such as thickening of the cusps (black arrow) in aortic valve stenosis

Differential Diagnosis

- ► Other causes of aortic stenosis
- ► Other aortic valve anomalies (e.g., unicuspid valve)

Teaching Points

- ► Associated with coarctation of the aorta, Williams syndrome, interrupted aortic arch, Turner syndrome (30% have bicuspid valves), LCA dominance
- ► Epidemiology: Most common congenital cardiac malformation (1%–2% of the population), autosomal dominant inheritance with incomplete penetrance, males > females (2:1)
- ► Presentation: Usually asymptomatic until complications develop
- ► Complications: Aortic valve stenosis, aortic regurgitation, endocarditis, aortic dilatation, aneurysm, dissection

Management

- ► Once diagnosed, serial imaging follow-up and antibiotic prophylaxis are recommended; screening of first-degree relatives is also advocated
- ► Aortic valve replacement (or a pulmonary autograft in pediatric patients) for severe valvular dysfunction, symptomatic patients, and/or patients with abnormal LV dimensions and function

Further Readings

Fedak PW et al. Clinical and pathophysiological implications of a bicuspid aortic valve. *Circulation.* 2002;106(8):900–904.
Yener N et al. Bicuspid aortic valve. *Ann Thorac Cardiovasc Surg.* 2002;8(5):264–267.

History

▶ None

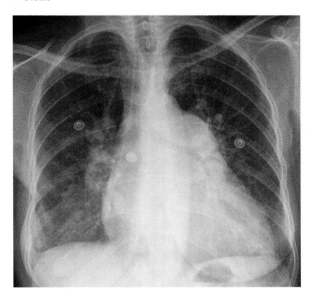

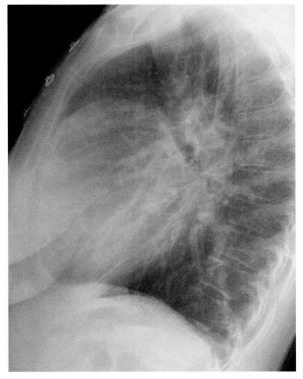

Case 85 Mitral Stenosis (CXR)

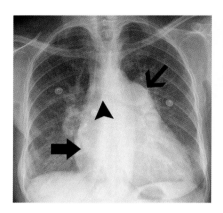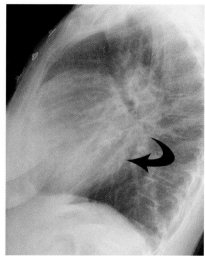

Findings

- ► CXR:
  - ▪ Frontal view: LA enlargement—double contour of the right heart border (block arrow), splaying of the carina (arrowhead), upward displacement of the left main bronchus, LA bulge (arrow)—followed by PA, RV, and RA enlargement, pulmonary edema
  - ▪ Lateral view: Posterior bulge of the LA (curved arrow)

Differential Diagnosis

- ► Cor triatriatum
- ► LA myxoma
- ► LA ball-valve thrombus
- ► Infective endocarditis

Teaching Points

- ► Gradual narrowing of the inlet valve orifice of the LV, resulting in obstruction of flow from the LA to the LV during diastole
- ► Etiology: Rheumatic heart disease (most common), severe mitral annular calcification, parachute mitral valve deformity
- ► Epidemiology: Females > males (2:1)
- ► Presentation: Dyspnea, fatigue, atrial arrhythmia
- ► Complications: Atrial fibrillation, LA thrombus, embolic event, pulmonary HTN, RV failure, tricuspid regurgitation, pulmonary regurgitation

Management

- ► Medical therapy (antibiotics, diuretics, dietary sodium restriction, nitrates, β-blocker, calcium channel blocker, anticoangulation) to reduce recurrence of rheumatic fever, prevent infective endocarditis, reduce cardiac preload, control arrhythmia, and prevent an embolic event
- ► Percutaneous balloon valvuloplasty is considered in patients with uncomplicated mitral stenosis; if not, valvotomy or mitral valve replacement can be considered

Further Reading

See Case 86: Mitral Stenosis (CT).

History

▶ None

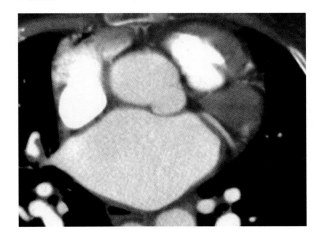

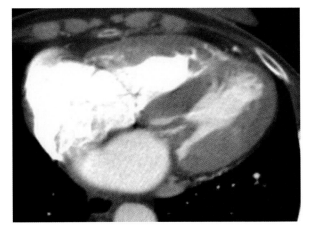

Case 86 Mitral Stenosis (CT)

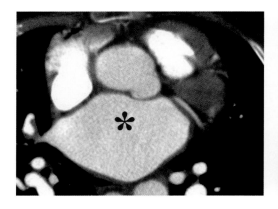 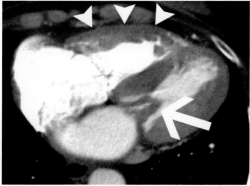

Findings

- ► CTA:
  - Funnel-shaped mitral valve (arrow), thickened and calcified leaflets, fusion of chordae tendinae
  - LA enlargement (asterisk) ± thrombus formation
  - Pulmonary edema, RV hypertrophy (arrowheads)
  - Cine: Restricted movement of the leaflets
- ► MR:
  - Thickening of mitral valve leaflets, LA enlargement
  - SSFP: Diastolic flow void across the stenosis, decreased excursion of valve cusps during the diastolic phase
  - Phase contrast: Increased flow velocity and flow gradient across the stenosis

Differential Diagnosis

- ► *See Case: Mitral Stenosis (CXR)*

Teaching Points

- ► *See Case 85: Mitral Stenosis (CXR)*

Management

- ► *See Case 85: Mitral Stenosis (CXR)*

Further Readings

Glockner JF et al. Evaluation of cardiac valvular disease with MR imaging: qualitative and quantitative techniques. *Radiographics*. 2003;23(1):e9.

Messika-Zeitoun D et al. Assessment of the mitral valve area in patients with mitral stenosis by multislice computed tomography. *J Am Coll Cardiol*. 2006;48(2):411–413.

Parker MS et al. Radiologic signs in thoracic imaging: case-based review and self-assessment module. *AJR Am J Roentgenol*. 2009;192(3)(suppl):S34–S48.

History

▶ None

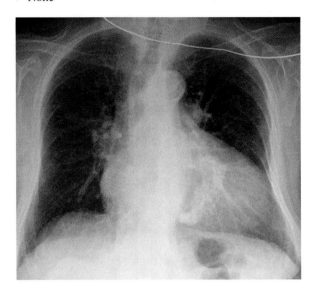

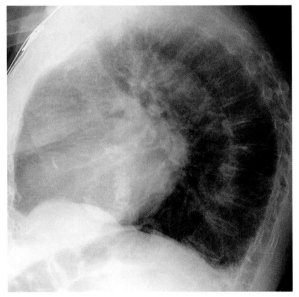

Case 87 Mitral Annular Calcification

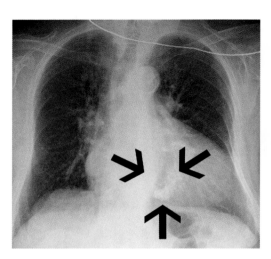 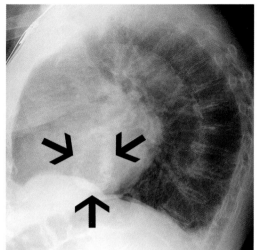

Findings

- ► CXR: Incomplete (J-, U-, reversed C-shaped) or complete (O-shaped) (arrows) band-like calcification of uniform radiopacity along the mitral annulus
- ► NECT: Dense calcification in the expected location of the posterior or entire mitral annulus
- ► MR: Signal dropout on all sequences around the mitral valve

Differential Diagnosis

- ► Caseous calcification of the mitral annulus
- ► Mitral valve calcificatìo n

Teaching Points

- ► Degenerative, commonly dystrophic, calcification of the mitral valve support ring
- ► Marker for severe CAD
- ► Risk factors: HTN, DM, mitral valve prolapse, aortic valve stenosis, end-stage renal disease, secondary hyperparathyroidism, hypercholesterolemia, atrial fibrillation
- ► Epidemiology: >40 years old (usually >65 years old), females > males
- ► Presentation: Usually asymptomatic unless massive
- ► Complications: Mitral stenosis, mitral regurgitation, infective endocarditis, atrial arrhythmias, heart block, embolic event

Management

- ► None; usually a benign incidental finding
- ► If clinically significant, mitral valve repair or replacement can be performed

Further Readings

Atar S et al. Mitral annular calcification: a marker of severe coronary artery disease in patients under 65 years old. *Heart.* 2003;89(2):161–164.

Fox CS et al. Framingham Heart Study. Mitral annular calcification predicts cardiovascular morbidity and mortality: the Framingham Heart Study. *Circulation.* 2003;107(11):1492–1496.

History

► None

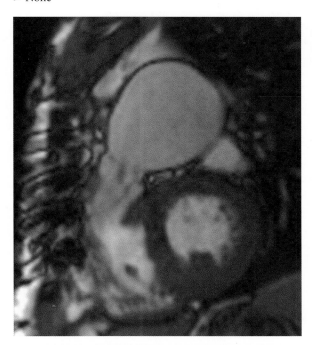

Figure 88-1   Steady-state free precession image in the diastolic phase

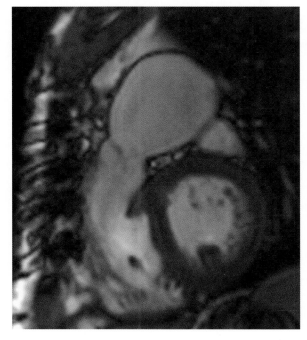

Figure 88-2   Steady-state free precession image in the diastolic phase

Case 88   Pulmonary Regurgitation

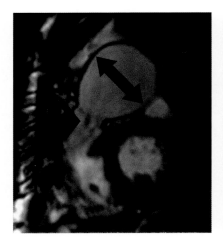 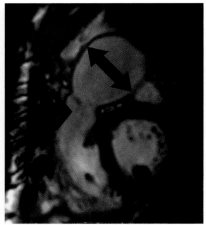

Findings

- ► CXR:
  - ▪ Frontal view: Dilated central PA, ± dilatation of the azygous vein and SVC
  - ▪ Lateral view: RV enlargement (filling of the retrosternal space)
- ► CTA:
  - ▪ Incomplete apposition of the cusps during diastole
  - ▪ Dilatation of the pulmonic ring and PA
  - ▪ Compensatory changes—RV dilatation and hypertrophy
- ► MR:
  - ▪ Malcoaptation of pulmonary valve cusps during diastole, RV dilatation and hypertrophy, dilated central PA (double arrows)
  - ▪ SSFP MR: Retrograde flow void in diastole across the incompletely coapted pulmonary valves (arrows)
  - ▪ Phase-contrast MR: Assess the RV EF and the volume of regurgitation

Differential Diagnosis

- ► Mitral stenosis
- ► Right heart failure

Teaching Points

- ► Poor coaptation of the pulmonary valve cusps allowing leakage of blood from the PA to the RV during diastole
- ► Volume overload causes RV, PA dilatation ± azygous vein and SVC dilatation
- ► Etiology: PA HTN, Marfan syndrome, rheumatic heart disease, endocarditis, carcinoid disease, surgical complication (e.g., TOF repair)
- ► Presentation: Usually asymptomatic; dyspnea on exertion
- ► Complication: Right heart failure

Management

- ► Treat the underlying etiology
- ► Usually benign; valve repair or replacement only with significant heart failure

Further Readings

Bouzas B et al. Pulmonary regurgitation: not a benign lesion. *Eur Heart J.* 2005;26(5):433–439.
Cawley PJ et al. Cardiovascular magnetic resonance imaging for valvular heart disease: technique and validation. *Circulation.* 2009;119(3):468–478.

History

▶ None

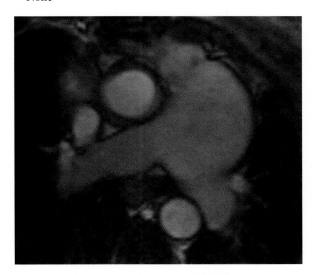

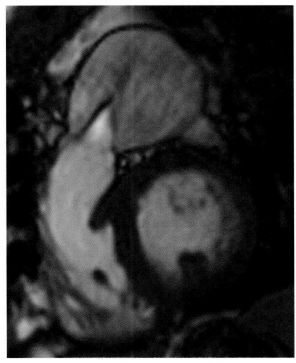

Case 89 Pulmonary Stenosis

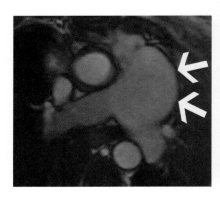
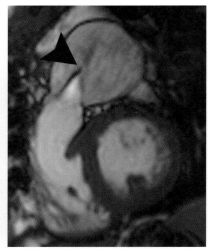

Findings

▶ CXR: Poststenotic dilatation of the left PA
▶ CTA:
  ▪ Thickening of the pulmonary valve cusps
  ▪ Compensatory changes—poststenotic enlargement of main and left PAs, RV hypertrophy with bowing of the interventricular septum to the left
  ▪ Cine: Decreased excursion of valve cusps during the systolic phase
▶ MR:
  ▪ Thickening of pulmonary valve cusps, compensatory changes (arrows)
  ▪ SSFP: Systolic flow void across the stenosis (arrowhead), decreased excursion of valve cusps during the systolic phase
  ▪ Phase contrast: Increased flow velocity and flow gradient across the stenosis

Differential Diagnosis

▶ Pulmonary HTN
▶ Idiopathic Dilatation of the PA

Teaching Points

▶ Gradual narrowing of the pulmonary valve area resulting in obstruction of flow from the RVOT to the PA during systole
▶ Right PA is usually not dilated since it is not exposed to the turbulent jet of the stenosis, a point of distinction from pulmonary HTN
▶ Etiology
  ▪ Congenital (and isolated) (95% of cases): TOF, pulmonary atresia
  ▪ Acquired: Rheumatic fever, metastatic carcinoid syndrome

Management

▶ Balloon valvuloplasty or surgical valvotomy for right heart failure or for a transvalvular pressure gradient >50 mmHg

Further Reading

Rebergen SA et al. Cine gradient-echo MR imaging and MR velocity mapping in the evaluation of congenital heart disease. *Radiographics.* 1996;16(3):467–481.

History

▶ None

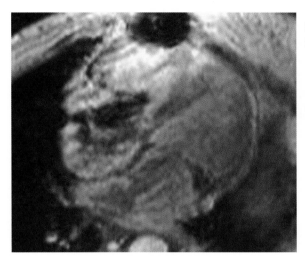

Figure 90-1   Bright blood image in the systolic phase

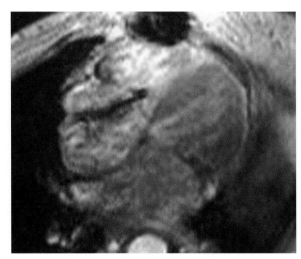

Figure 90-2   Bright blood image in the systolic phase

Case 90 Tricuspid Regurgitation

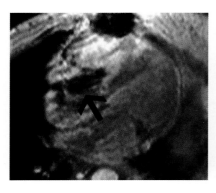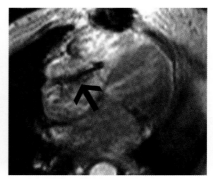

Findings

- ► CXR:
  - ▪ Frontal view: Prominent RA and RV, distention of the SVC and the azygous vein
  - ▪ Lateral view: Filling of the retrosternal clear space, distended IVC
- ► CTA/MRI:
  - ▪ Malcoaptation of tricuspid leaflets during systole
  - ▪ Dilated RA and RV, with the RV displaced to the left and the interventricular septum bowed to the left (cor pulmonale), distended SVC, azygous vein, IVC, and hepatic veins with systolic reflux of contrast
  - ▪ Findings of the underlying etiology (e.g., emphysema, pulmonary HTN)
  - ▪ SSFP MR: Retrograde flow void in systole (arrows) across the incompletely coapted tricuspid valves

Differential Diagnosis

- ► Dilated CM
- ► Ebstein anomaly

Teaching Points

- ► Tricuspid valve apparatus has three leaflets (septal, anterior, and posterior), papillary muscles, chordae tendinae, and an annulus
- ► Usually thinner than the mitral valve due to lower right-sided pressures
- ► Etiology :
  - ▪ Primary: Rheumatic heart disease, infectious endocarditis, MI, metastatic carcinoid syndrome, trauma, Marfan syndrome
  - ▪ Secondary: More common; elevated PA pressure (e.g., left heart failure, pulmonary HTN, or COPD) resulting in dilatation of the RV and the tricuspid annulus with stretching of the leaflets
- ► Presentation: Usually asymptomatic; elevated jugular venous pressure, peripheral edema, right upper quadrant discomfort, fatigue, ascites, cardiac cirrhosis

Management

- ► Medical therapy (diuretics) to reduce the cardiac preload ± afterload
- ► Annuloplasty or valve replacement is rarely indicated since most cases are the result of RV or tricuspid annular dilatation

Further Readings

Boxt LM. Radiology of the right ventricle. *Radiol Clin North Am.* 1999;37(2):379–400.
Shah PM et al. Tricuspid valve disease. *Curr Probl Cardiol.* 2008;33(2):47–84.

History

▶ None

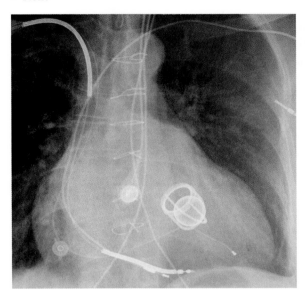

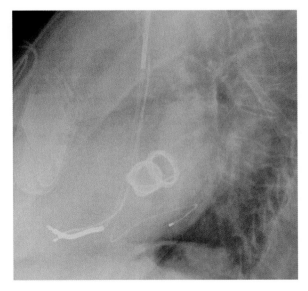

Case 91 Valvular Prosthesis

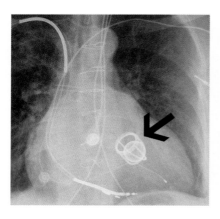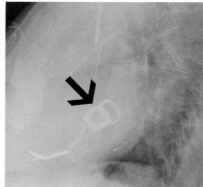

Findings

- ▶ CXR: Type of prosthetic valve, such as ball-in-cage valve (arrows)
- ▶ Fluoroscopy: Traditionally used to assess the function of the valve
- ▶ CTA/MR: Assess the function of the valve, ± prosthetic complications
  - ▪ CTA: Mechanical leaflet motion, opening angle

Differential Diagnosis

- ▶ Aortic calcifications
- ▶ Annuloplasty ring

Teaching Points

- ▶ Most commonly performed for the aortic and mitral valves
- ▶ Two main types:
  - ▪ Biological
    - ◆ Major types: Allograft, xenograft (e.g., porcine, bovine, equine); usually mounted on a support frame
    - ◆ Limited durability (15 years)
    - ◆ Preferred for tricuspid valve replacement due to the higher risk of thrombus formation
  - ▪ Mechanical
    - ◆ Major types: Ball-in-cage, tilting disk, bileaflet
    - ◆ Longer durability (20–30 years)
    - ◆ Two times the complication rate (2%–4%) as biological valves
- ▶ Complications: "Frozen" leaflets from the thrombus or pannus, valve dehiscence, hemorrhage, pseudoaneurysm, infectious endocarditis, paravalvular abscess

Management

- ▶ Mechanical prosthetic valves require lifelong anticoagulation therapy
- ▶ Biological prosthetic valves only require short-term anticoagulation therapy after implantation (3 months)

Further Readings

Gilkeson RC et al. MDCT evaluation of aortic valvular disease. *AJR Am J Roentgenol.* 2006;186(2):350–360.

Landay MJ et al. Cardiac valve reconstruction and replacement: a brief review. *Radiographics.* 1992;12(4):659–671.

Steiner RM et al. The radiology of cardiac valve prostheses. *Radiographics.* 1988;8(2):277–298.

History

► None

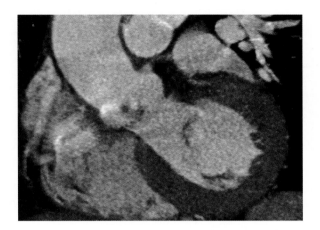

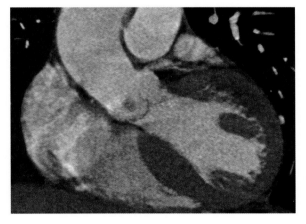

Case 92 Papillary Fibroelastoma

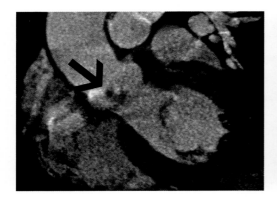 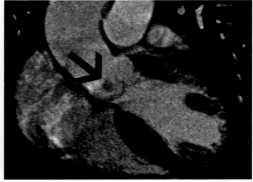

Findings

- Location: Aortic valve (most common), mitral valve (second most common)
- CTA/MR: Small (<1.5 cm), pedunculated mass (arrows) arising from the valvular or endocardial surface
  - T2WI MR: Hypointense mass
  - SSFP MR: Turbulent blood flow

Differential Diagnosis

- Thrombus
- Atrial myxoma

Teaching Points

- Epidemiology:
  - Second most common primary benign cardiac tumor; myxoma is the most common
  - Most common primary valvular tumor
  - Males = females; mean age, 60 years
- Presentation: Usually asymptomatic; chest pain, dyspnea, syncope, blindness
- Complications: Cerebral stroke or transient ischemic attack, other embolic events (e.g., MI, pulmonary embolism), sudden death

Management

- None; usually an incidental finding at autopsy
- If it is clinically significant, surgical resection ± valve repair, or valve replacement can be performed

Further Readings

Burke A et al. Cardiac tumours: an update: Cardiac tumours. *Heart*. 2008;94(1):117–123.
Gowda RM et al. Cardiac papillary fibroelastoma: a comprehensive analysis of 725 cases. *Am Heart J*. 2003;146(3):404–410.
Grebenc ML et al. Primary cardiac and pericardial neoplasms: radiologic–pathologic correlation. *Radiographics*. 2000;20(4):1073–1103.

History

▶ A 45-year-old male with a history of gunshot wounds and intravenous drug use

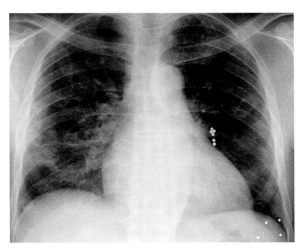

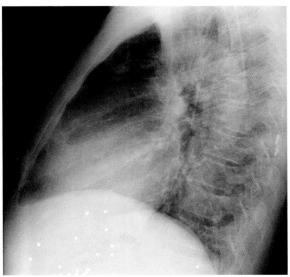

Case 93 Infective Endocarditis (CXR)

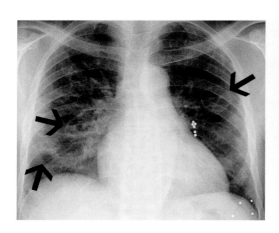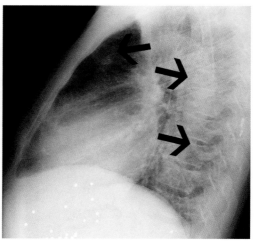

Findings

▶ CXR: Secondary signs from septic emboli, such as multiple nodular opacities and cavitations bilaterally (arrows), pleural effusion, large RA (from tricuspid regurgitation)

Differential Diagnosis

▶ Pulmonary metastases (e.g., squamous cell carcinoma)
▶ Granulomatous lung disease (e.g., tuberculosis, sarcoidosis)

Teaching Points

▶ Most common microorganisms include the following:
  ▪ Bacterial: Alpha-hemolytic *Streptococcus, Staphylococcus aureus, Enterococcus, Pseudomonas*
  ▪ Fungal: *Candida*
▶ Risk factors: Rheumatic valve disease, intravenous drug use, poor dental hygiene, long-term hemodialysis, DM, mitral valve prolapse, valvular prosthesis
  ▪ Certain risk factors may predispose to involvement of specific valves (e.g., intravenous drug use predominantly affects the tricuspid valve)
▶ Epidemiology: Incidence of 1.7–6.2/100,000 persons per year in developed countries
▶ Presentation: Fever of unknown origin, changing heart murmur, Osler's nodes, splinter hemorrhage
▶ Complications: Perivalvular abscess, pseudoaneurysm, valvular heart disease, septic embolic events

Management

▶ Medical therapy with long-term intravenous antibiotics
▶ Surgical debridement and valve replacement is reserved for patients with failed antibiotic therapy

Further Reading

See Case 94: Infective Endocarditis (CT).

History

▶ A 45-year-old male with a history of intravenous drug use presents with fever

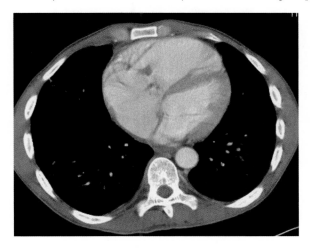

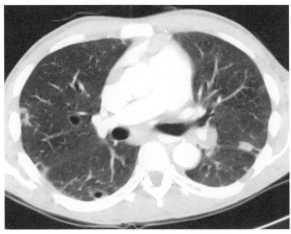

Case 94 Infective Endocarditis (CT)

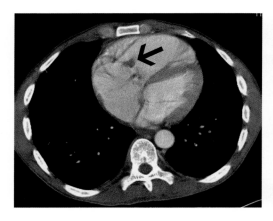 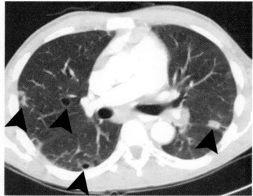

Findings

▶ CTA/MR:
  - Irregular mass arising from a valve (arrow) or, less frequently, from other cardiac structures
  - Particularly useful in evaluation of associated complications such as perivalvular abscess or pulmonary septic emboli (arrowheads)
  - Cine: Mobile mass
  - T1+Gad MR: Enhancement of the mass

Differential Diagnosis

▶ Other causes of valvular heart disease (e.g., rheumatic heart disease, age-related degeneration)

Teaching Points

▶ *See Case: Infective Endocarditis (CXR)*

Management

▶ *See Case 93: Infective Endocarditis (CXR)*

Further Readings

Akins EW et al. Perivalvular pseudoaneurysm complicating bacterial endocarditis: MR detection in five cases. *AJR Am J Roentgenol.* 1991;156(6):1155–1158.

Chen JJ et al. CT angiography of the cardiac valves: normal, diseased, and postoperative appearances. *Radiographics.* 2009;29(5):1393–1412.

Pollak Y et al. *Staphylococcus aureus* endocarditis of the aortic valve diagnosed on MR imaging. *AJR Am J Roentgenol.* 2002;179(6):1647.

History

▶ A 45-year-old male with nonexertional stabbing chest pain

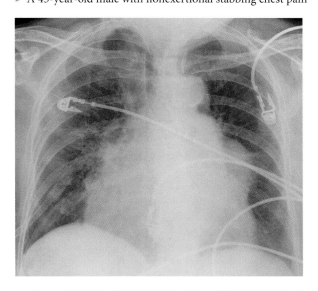

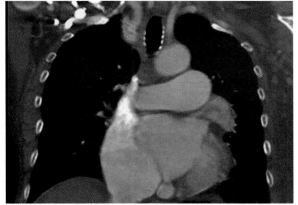

Case 95 Congenital Absence of the Pericardium

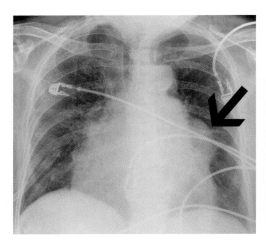
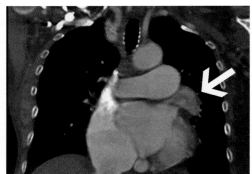

Findings

- ▶ Two types: Complete or partial; the partial left-sided defect is more common
- ▶ CXR: Frontal view: Levoposition of the heart, flattening and elongation of the left heart border, lucency between the aorta and PA or between the diaphragm and the base of the heart, prominence of the LA appendage
- ▶ CT/MR: Interposition of lung tissue between the aorta and PA or between the diaphragm and base of the heart, leftward cardiac displacement, bulging of the LA appendage (arrows)
  - ▪ Cine: Substantial movement of the LV apex, large variation between end-systolic and end-diastolic heart volume

Differential Diagnosis

- ▶ Causes of RV enlargement (e.g., pulmonary stenosis)
- ▶ Pericardial cyst
- ▶ Thymic mass (e.g., thymic cyst, thymolipoma)
- ▶ Pericardial effusion
- ▶ Loculated pleural effusion
- ▶ LV aneurysm

Teaching Points

- ▶ Epidemiology: Males > females (3:1)
- ▶ Usually occurs in isolation but can be associated with ASD, PDA, mitral stenosis, or TOF
- ▶ Presentation: Usually asymptomatic; nonexertional stabbing chest pain mimicking CAD, incomplete right bundle branch block (RBBB) with poor R-wave progression on the ECG
- ▶ Complications: In the partial absence of the pericardium, herniation and strangulation of a cardiac chamber, especially the LA appendage, can occur

Management

- ▶ None; usually a benign congenital finding noted incidentally at cardiac surgery
- ▶ Surgical pericardectomy or pericardioplasty is only needed to treat symptomatic patients or patients who present with complications

Further Readings

Gatzoulis MA et al. Isolated congenital absence of the pericardium: clinical presentation, diagnosis, and management. *Ann Thorac Surg.* 2000;69(4):1209–1215.

Gehlmann HR et al. Symptomatic congenital complete absence of the left pericardium. Case report and review of the literature. *Eur Heart J.* 1989;10(7):670–675.

Psychidis-Papakyritsis P et al. Functional MRI of congenital absence of the pericardium. *AJR Am J Roentgenol.* 2007;189(6):W312–W314.

History

▶ A 50-year-old male with shortness of breath

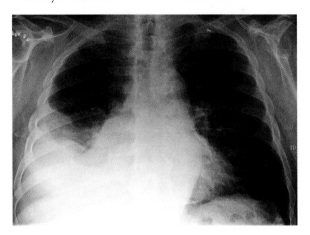

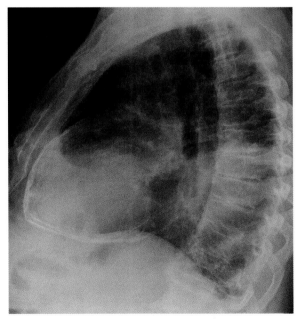

Case 96 Pericardial Calcification (CXR)

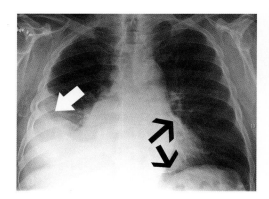
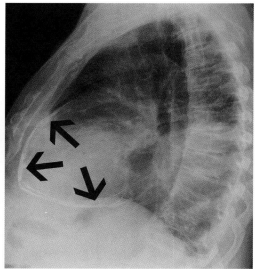

Findings

- ► CXR
- ► Calcification over the anterior and diaphragmatic aspects of the heart (arrows; best seen on the lateral view), with the AV groove and RA frequently involved (the LA is usually spared)
- ► ± associated findings or complications, such as pleural effusion (block arrow) in heart failure

Differential Diagnosis

- ► Myocardial calcification (e.g., chronic MI, LV aneurysm)
- ► Teratoma
- ► Coronary artery calcification
- ► Mitral annulus calcification

Teaching Points

- ► Pericardial calcification can be differentiated from myocardial calcification by the involvement of the AV groove, affecting mainly the right heart and sparing the LA and apex
- ► Etiology: Infectious pericarditis (e.g., coxsackievirus, influenza, histoplasmosis, tuberculosis), uremic pericarditis, connective tissue disease (e.g., systemic lupus erythematosus), rheumatic heart disease, hemopericardium (e.g., trauma, cardiac surgery)
- ► Associated with constrictive pericarditis (>50% of patients)
- ► Presentation: Nonspecific; jugular venous distention, Kussmaul's sign
- ► Complication: CHF

Management

- ► Surgical stripping of the pericardium if clinically indicated

Further Reading

See Case 97: Pericardial Calcification (CT).

History

▸ A 50-year-old male with shortness of breath

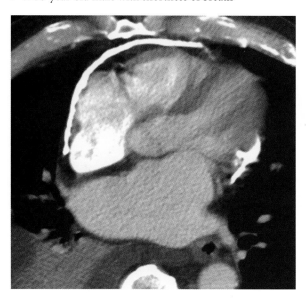

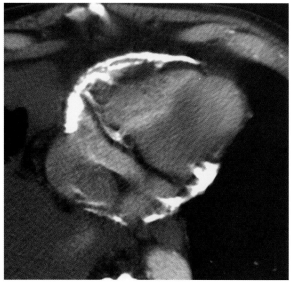

Case 97 Pericardial Calcification (CT)

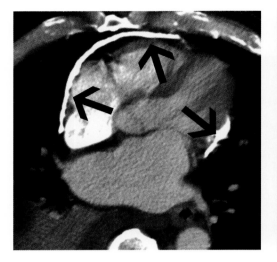 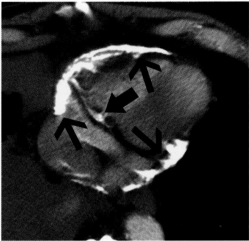

Findings

▶ CT:
- Calcification (arrows) usually affecting the right side of the heart, including the RV, AV groove (block arrow), and RA
- Calcification can also be diffuse, but it spares the LA and left apex
- Associated findings or complications, such as a tubular ventricular configuration in constrictive pericarditis

▶ MR:
- Circumscribed signal void on all sequences
- T1WI: Surrounded by high-signal epicardial fat

Differential Diagnosis

▶ Pericardial effusion/tamponade
▶ Myocardial calcification (e.g., chronic MI)
▶ Restrictive CM (e.g., amyloidosis, sarcoidosis)
▶ Pericardial metastases

Teaching Points

▶ *See Case 96: Pericardial Calcification (CXR)*

Management

▶ *See Case 96: Pericardial Calcification (CXR)*

Further Readings

MacGregor JH et al. The radiographic distinction between pericardial and myocardial calcifications. *AJR Am J Roentgenol.* 1987;148(4):675–677.

Olson MC et al. Computed tomography and magnetic resonance imaging of the pericardium. *Radiographics.* 1989;9(4):633–634.

Rozenshtein A et al. Plain-film diagnosis of pericardial disease. *Semin Roentgenol.* 1999;34(3):195–204.

History

▶ None

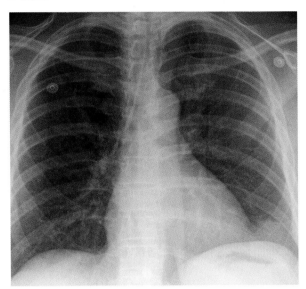

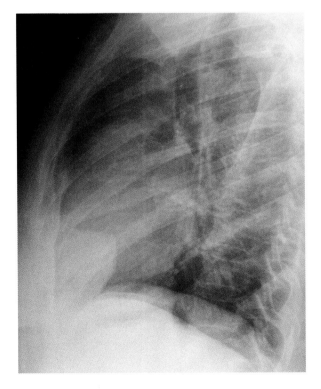

Case 98 Pericardial Cyst (CXR)

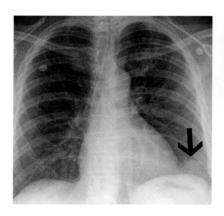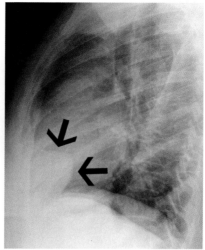

Findings

▸ Location: Right > left anterior cardiophrenic space; can be located throughout the mediastinum

▸ CXR: Mass with well-defined borders occupying the cardiophrenic space (see arrows)

Differential Diagnosis

▸ Bronchogenic cyst
▸ Loculated pleural effusion
▸ Pericardial fat pad
▸ Enlarged percardial lymph nodes
▸ Thymic tumors (e.g., thymic cyst, thymolipoma)
▸ Hydatid cyst
▸ Pericardial hematoma
▸ Morgagni hernia

Teaching Points

▸ Lesion tends to change in shape or size with respiration or changes in body positioning
▸ 5%–10% of all mediastinal tumors
▸ Etiology: Congenital
▸ Presentation: Usually asymptomatic, although it can manifest as a palpable mass, dyspnea, retrosternal discomfort, or arrhythmia

Management

▸ None; usually a benign finding noted incidentally on imaging
▸ If it is clinically significant, surgical resection can be performed

Further Reading

See Case 99: Pericardial Cyst (CT).

History

▶ None

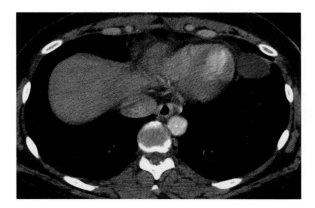

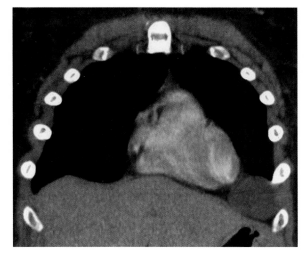

Case 99 Pericardial Cyst (CT)

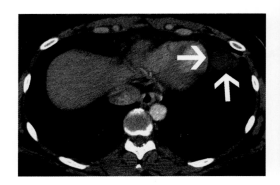
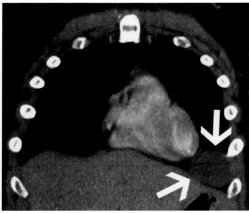

Findings

- ▶ Location: Right > left anterior cardiophrenic space; can be located throughout the mediastinum
- ▶ CT:
  - ▪ NECT: Fluid-filled lesion (0–20 HU; may have higher HU if the lesion contains proteinaceous fluid) with well-defined borders and thin, smooth walls (arrows), usually without internal septa
  - ▪ CECT: No enhancement
- ▶ MR:
  - ▪ T1WI: Mass with homogeneous low to intermediate signal intensity (may have higher signal intensity if the mass contains proteinaceous fluid)
  - ▪ T2WI: Mass with homogeneous high signal intensity
  - ▪ T1+Gad: No enhancement after gadolinium contrast administration

Differential Diagnosis

- ▶ Bronchogenic cyst
- ▶ Thymic cyst
- ▶ Hydatid cyst
- ▶ Loculated pleural effusion
- ▶ Pericardial hematoma

Teaching Points

- ▶ *See Case 98: Pericardial Cyst (CXR)*

Management

- ▶ *See Case 98: Pericardial Cyst (CXR)*

Further Readings

Dursun M et al. Cardiac hydatid disease: CT and MRI findings. *AJR Am J Roentgenol.* 2008;190(1): 226–232.

Oyama N et al. Computed tomography and magnetic resonance imaging of the pericardium: anatomy and pathology. *Magn Reson Med Sci.* 2004;3(3):145–152.

Pineda V et al. Lesions of the cardiophrenic space: findings at cross-sectional imaging. *Radiographics.* 2007;27(1):19–32.

History

▶ A 54-year-old male with chest and back pain

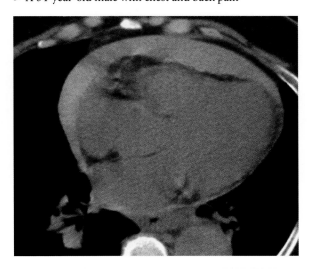

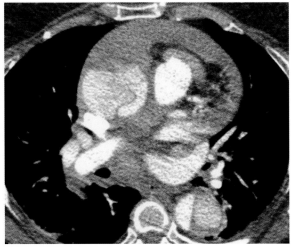

Case 100 Hemopericardium

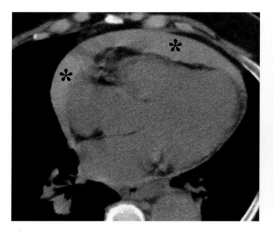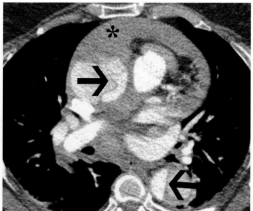

Findings

- CXR:
    - Frontal view: "Water-bottle" configuration (*See Case 101: Pericardial Effusion [CXR]*)
    - Lateral view: "Epicardial fat pad" sign
- CT: Hyperdense fluid (>35 HU) surrounding the heart (asterisks); attenuation decreases with age; findings of the underlying etiology, such as an intramural flap (arrows) in aortic dissection
- MR: Heterogeneous signal intensity that varies with age and depends on the sequences acquired

Differential Diagnosis

- Pericarditis (e.g., infectious, uremic)
- Other causes of pericardial effusion
- Coronary artery aneurysm

Teaching Points

- Etiology: Trauma (e.g., cardiac chamber rupture, aortic root rupture, coronary artery laceration), aortic dissection, MI, iatrogenic (e.g., endovascular radiofrequency ablation of atrial fibrillation, anticoagulation therapy), malignancy (e.g., metastases, angiosarcoma)
- Presentation: Asymptomatic to mild symptoms (e.g., tachycardia, dyspnea) to total cardiovascular collapse
- Complications: Pericardial tamponade, constrictive pericarditis

Management

- Surgical or medical therapy is required, depending on the etiology

Further Readings

Krejci CS et al. Hemopericardium: an emergent finding in a case of blunt cardiac injury. *AJR Am J Roentgenol.* 2000;175(1):250.

Olson MC et al. Computed tomography and magnetic resonance imaging of the pericardium. *Radiographics.* 1989;9(4):633–634.

History

▸ None

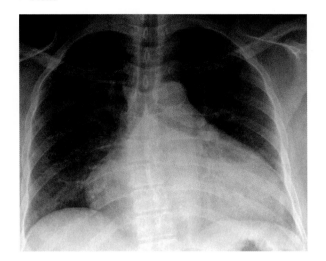

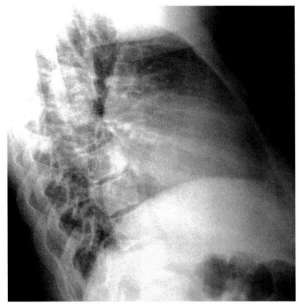

Case 101 Pericardial Effusion (CXR)

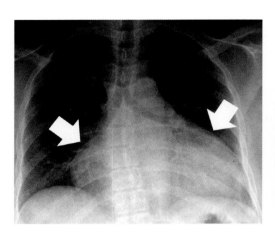 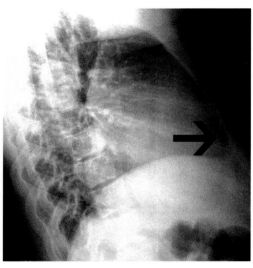

Findings

- CXR:
  - Frontal view: "Water-bottle" configuration (symmetrically enlarged cardiopericardial silhouette assuming the shape of a flask or water bottle) (block arrows)
  - Lateral view: "Epicardial fat pad" sign (fluid between the retrosternal fat and the epicardial fat accentuates the epicardial fat pad) (arrow)

Differential Diagnosis

- Causes of cardiomegaly (e.g., left heart failure, dilated CM)
- Pericardial cyst (if loculated)

Teaching Points

- Etiology: CHF, renal insufficiency, connective tissue disease (e.g., systemic lupus erythematosus), infection (e.g., coxsackievirus, HIV, tuberculosis), malignancy (e.g., lung or breast carcinoma, lymphoma), MI (Dressler syndrome), hypothyroidism, trauma, iatrogenic
- Presentation: Asymptomatic to chest pain, dyspnea, cough. Ewart's sign (dullness to percussion, increased fremitus and bronchial breathing beneath the angle of the left scapula found with large pericardial effusions)
- Complications: Pericardial tamponade, constrictive pericarditis

Management

- Treat the underlying etiology
- If the patient is symptomatic, pericardiocentesis or pericardial window surgery can be performe d

Further Reading

See Case 102: Pericardial Effusion (CT).

History

▶ None

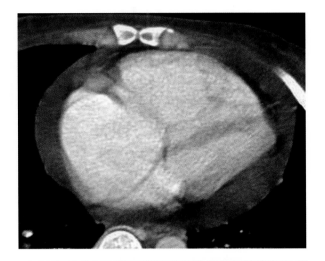

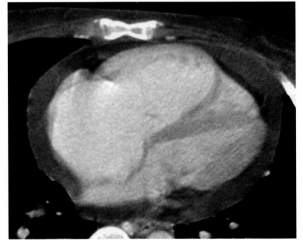

Case 102 Pericardial Effusion (CT)

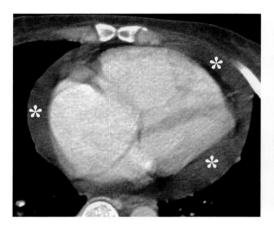 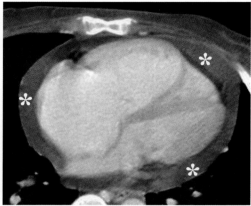

Findings

▶ CT/MR:

  ▪ Fluid-filled space surrounding the heart (asterisks); accumulation first occurs posterior to the left side of the heart (if the patient is supine)

  ▪ Attenuation/intensity of the fluid will vary, depending on the type of fluid (e.g., serous, blood, chyle, or purulent)

  ▪ Findings of the underlying etiology (e.g., irregularly thickened pericardium or pleural nodularity suggests malignancy)

Differential Diagnosis

▶ Pericardial tamponade

▶ Pericardial metastases

▶ Pericardial cyst (if loculated)

Teaching Points

▶ *See Case 101: Pericardial Effusion (CXR)*

Management

▶ *See Case 101: Pericardial Effusion (CXR)*

Further Readings

Breen JF. Imaging of the pericardium. *J Thorac Imaging*. 2001;16(1):47–54.

Silverman PM et al. Computed tomography of the abnormal pericardium. *AJR Am J Roentgenol*. 1983;140(6):1125–1129.

Wang ZJ et al. CT and MR imaging of pericardial disease. *Radiographics*. 2003;23 Spec No:S167–S180.

History

▸ A 38-year-old female with a history of HIV and lymphoma presents with dyspnea

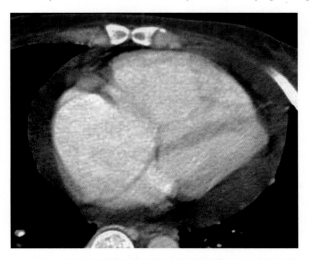

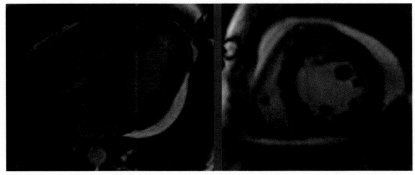

Figure 103-2   Four-chamber (left) and two-chamber (right) bright blood images in the diastolic phase

Case 103 Pericardial Tamponade

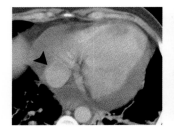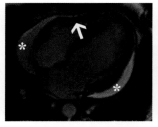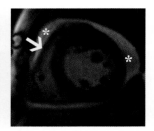

Findings

- ► CXR: Rapidly enlarging cardiopericardial silhouette, water-bottle configuration of the cardiopericardial silhouette ± epicardial fat pad sign
- ► CT/MR:
  - ▪ Fluid-filled pericardial space (asterisks) with varying attenuation/intensity
  - ▪ Flattening of the lateral wall of the RV (arrows) or concave RV deformity
  - ▪ Angulation or bowing of the interventricular septum to the LV
  - ▪ Enlarged SVC, IVC (arrowhead), hepatic veins, renal veins
  - ▪ Reflux of contrast within the IVC and azygos vein
  - ▪ Findings of the underlying etiology (e.g., aortic dissection)
  - ▪ Cine: Diastoic septal bounce (paradoxical motion of the septum)

Differential Diagnosis

- ► Causes of cardiomegaly (for CXR findings)
- ► Pericardial effus ion without tamponade

Teaching Points

- ► Etiology:
  - ▪ Accumulation of serous fluid, pus, blood, gas, or neoplastic tissue within the intrapericardial space resulting in filling restriction of the cardiac chambers with reduced cardiac output
  - ▪ Trauma, MI, aortic dissection, aortic or coronary artery aneurysm rupture, iatrogenic (e.g., thrombolytic therapy), malignancy (e.g., lymphoma)
- ► Presentation: Dyspnea, tachycardia, hypotension, jugular venous distention, soft or muffled heart sounds, pulsus paradoxus

Management

- ► Pericardiocentesis or surgical drainage are the treatments of choice
- ► Pericardial sclerosis and balloon pericardiotomy are used in recurrent cases

Further Readings

Little WC et al. Pericardial disease. *Circulation.* 2006;113(12):1622–1632.
Restrepo CS et al. Imaging findings in cardiac tamponade with emphasis on CT. *Radiographics.* 2007;27(6):1595–1610.

History

▸ A 45-year-old male after a motor vehicle collision

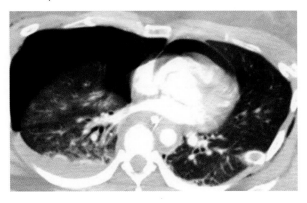

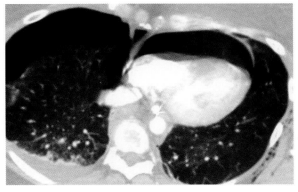

Case 104 Pneumopericardium

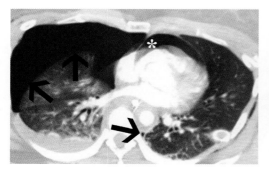 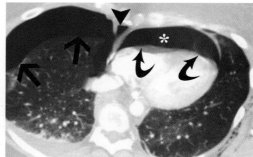

Findings

- ► CXR:
    - ▪ Radiolucent band of air partially or completely surrounding the heart ("halo" sign); the band is curved and sharply marginated by the pericardial sac
    - ▪ Lucency does not extend into the upper mediastinum or neck
    - ▪ Decubitus view: Gas collection shifts readily with altered patient position
    - ▪ Associated findings or complications, such as the "small heart" sign (significant decrease in the size of the cardiopericardial silhouette) in tension pneumopericardium
- ► CT: Air-filled pericardial cavity (asterisks), ± associated findings, such as pneumothorax (arrows) and pneumomediastinum (arrowhead), ± associated complications, such as a flattened anterior surface of the heart (curved arrows) in cardiac tamponade

Differential Diagnosis

- ► Pneumomediastinum
- ► Medial pneumothorax
- ► Pneumatocele
- ► Subcutaneous emphysema

Teaching Points

- ► Etiology: Trauma, iatrogenic (e.g., mechanical ventilation), pulmonary aspergillosis or tuberculosis, infectious pericarditis, severe asthma, congenital
- ► Associated with pneumomedastinum, pneumothorax
- ► Presentation: Chest pain, dyspnea, cyanosis, hypotension, tachycardia, pulsus paradoxus, Hamman's sign
- ► Complications: Tension pneumopericardium, cardiac tamponade

Management

- ► Pericardiocentesis ± drainage catheter placement

Further Readings

Bejvan SM et al. Pneumomediastinum: old signs and new signs. *AJR Am J Roentgenol.* 1996;166(5):1041–1048.

Mirvis SE et al. Posttraumatic tension pneumopericardium: the "small heart" sign. *Radiology.* 1986;158(3):663–669.

Restrepo CS et al. Imaging findings in cardiac tamponade with emphasis on CT. *Radiographics.* 2007;27(6):1595–1610.

History

▶ A 36-year-old male presents with recurrent pericardial effusions and dyspnea

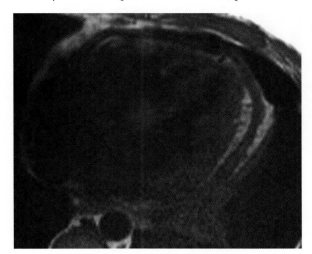

Figure 105-1   T1-weighted

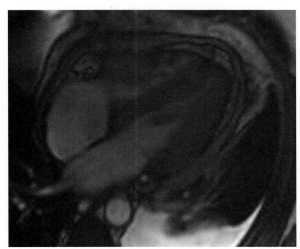

Figure 105-2   Bright blood

Case 105 Constrictive Pericarditis

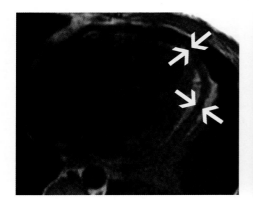 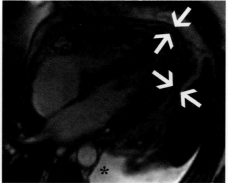

Findings

- ► CXR: ± Pericardial calcification (*See Case 96: Pericardial Calcification [CXR]*)
- ► CT/MR:
  - ▪ Abnormal pericardial thickening (≥4 mm) (arrows); may be limited to the right side of the heart or the right AV groove, ± pericardial effusion (attenuation/intensity depends on the content of the effusion)
  - ▪ Pericardial calcification (hyperdense on NECT, signal void on MR) (*See Case 97: Pericardial Calcification [CT]*)
  - ▪ Tubular configuration of the RV, sigmoid-shaped or prominent leftward convexity of the ventricular septum
  - ▪ CECT/T1+Gad: ± Pericardial enhancement
  - ▪ Cine: Diastolic septal bounce (paradoxical motion of the septum)
  - ▪ Associated complications, such as enlarged IVC, pleural effusions (asterisk)

Differential Diagnosis

- ► Restrictive CM (e.g., amyloidosis, sarcoidosis)
- ► Cardiac tamponade
- ► Pleural effusion
- ► Pericarditis without constriction (e.g., infectious, uremic)
- ► Pericardial calcification without constriction
- ► Myocardial calcification

Teaching Points

- ► Diagnosis is based on the symptoms of constriction; imaging is an adjunct
- ► Etiology: Iatrogenic (e.g., cardiac surgery, radiation), infection (e.g., tuberculosis, coxsackievirus), connective tissue disease, uremia, malignancy, idiopathic
- ► Presentation: Dyspnea, orthopnea, jugular venous distention, Kussmaul's sign
- ► Complications: CHF

Management

- ► Acute: Medical therapy (anti-inflammatory agents, colchicine, steroids)
- ► Chronic: Surgical (pericardial decortication)

Further Readings

Little WC et al. Pericardial disease. *Circulation.* 2006;113(12):1622–1632.
Masui T et al. Constrictive pericarditis and restrictive cardiomyopathy: evaluation with MR imaging. *Radiology.* 1992;182(2):369–373.
Wang ZJ et al. CT and MR imaging of pericardial disease. *Radiographics.* 2003;23 Spec No:S167–S180.

History

▶ A 66-year-old male presents with fever and a pericardial rub

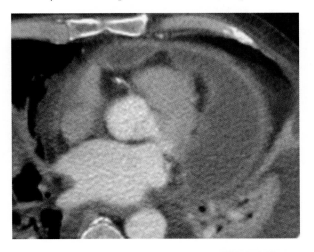

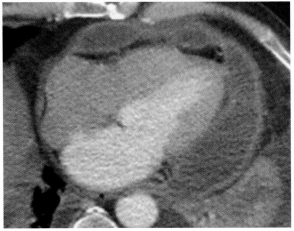

Case 106 Infectious Pericarditis

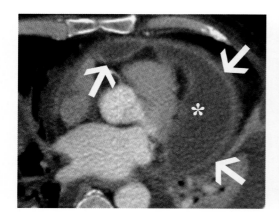
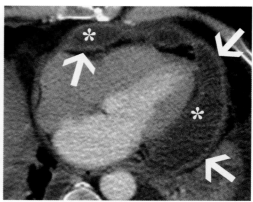

Findings

- ► CXR: "Water bottle" configuration, "epicardial fat pad" sign (*See Case 101: Pericardial Effusion [CXR]*)
- ► CT/MR: Diffuse or loculated pericardial effusion (asterisks) ± thickening (arrows), septation(s), and/or gas; enlarged lymph nodes
  - CECT/T1+Gad: Enhancement of the pericardium (arrows) ± septation(s)

Differential Diagnosis

- ► Other causes of pericarditis (e.g., uremia, connective tissue disease, MI, malignancy, trauma, iatrogenic)
- ► Mediastinal abscess
- ► Pericardial cyst (if loculated)

Teaching Points

- ► Etiology: Coxsackievirus, influenza, HIV, histoplasmosis, tuberculosis (as in this case)
- ► Presentation: Chest pain worsened with inspiration and relieved by sitting forward, dyspnea, pericardial friction rub
- ► Complications: Pericardial calcification, constrictive pericarditis, pericardial tamponade

Management

- ► Medical therapy (antibiotics) ± pericardiocentesis with possible drain catheter placement to culture and drain the purulent content

Further Readings

Kim HY et al. Thoracic sequelae and complications of tuberculosis. *Radiographics.* 2001;21(4):839–858; discussion 859–860.

Little WC et al. Pericardial disease. *Circulation.* 2006;113(12):1622–1632.

Wang ZJ et al. CT and MR imaging of pericardial disease. *Radiographics.* 2003;23 Spec No:S167–S180.

Part 11   Support Devices

History

▶ A 60-year-old male with dyspnea

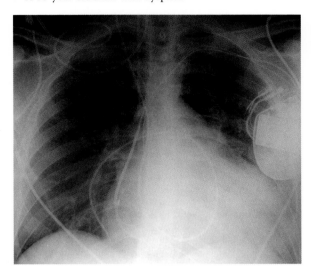

Figure 107-1 Day 1 in the intensive care unit

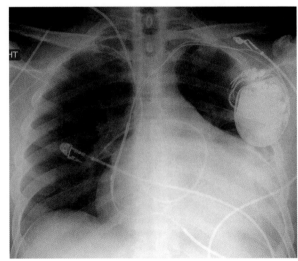

Figure 107-2 Day 2 in the intensive care unit

Case 107 Pulmonary Artery Catheter

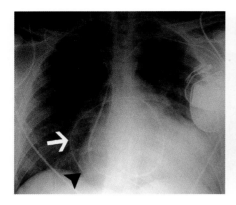 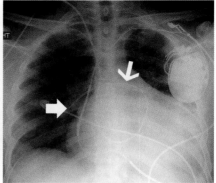

Findings

▶ CXR:
  ▪ Access obtained from the subclavian, internal jugular (as in this case), antecubital, or femoral vein
  ▪ Proper position:
    ◆ Catheter (arrows) traverses the SVC/IVC, RA, and RV
    ◆ Distal tip within the main PA, or either within the right PA (block arrow) or left PA
    ◆ When measuring pulmonary capillary wedge pressure, the catheter should be placed in the lower lobe (zone 3 of West)
  ▪ Improper position:
    ◆ Distal tip (arrowhead) is proximal to the main PA or distal (>2 cm lateral to the hilum) to either the right PA or the left PA
    ◆ In other tributary vessels (e.g., internal mammary or azygous vein)

Differential Diagnosis

▶ Other types of catheter (e.g., central venous line)
▶ External wire/tube(s)

Teaching Points

▶ *Also known as a Swan-Ganz catheter*
▶ Made up of two or three lumens with an inflatable balloon close to the tip
▶ Catheter used to monitor circulatory hemodynamics, including pressure in the LA and pulmonary capillary wedge pressure
▶ Complication: Lung infarction, PA pseudoaneurysm ± hemorrhage, arrhythmia, RV perforation, infection, thromboembolism, looping, pinching, or fragmentation of the catheter, pneumothorax or nerve injury during placement

Management

▶ If pseudoaneurysm develops, coil embolization is the treatment of choice

Further Readings

Ferretti GR et al. False aneurysm of the pulmonary artery induced by a Swan-Ganz catheter: clinical presentation and radiologic management. *AJR Am J Roentgenol.* 1996;167(4):941–945.
Hunter TB et al. Medical devices of the chest. *Radiographics.* 2004;24(6):1725–1746.

History

▸ A 64-year-old female with a history of arrhythmia

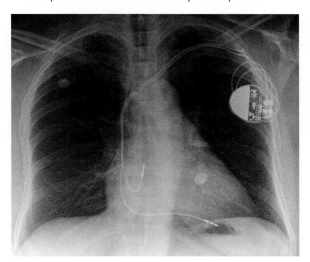

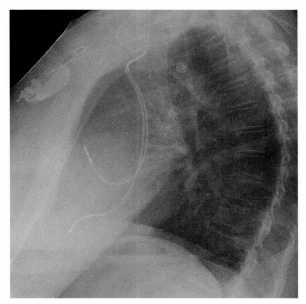

Case 108   Permanent Cardiac Pacemaker

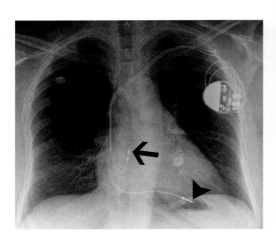
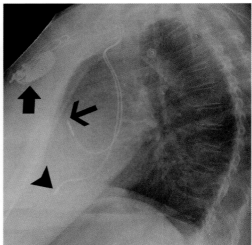

Findings

- ► CXR:
    - ▪ Access from the left or right subclavian vein
    - ▪ Pacemaker generator is commonly placed in the infraclavicular region (block arrow)
    - ▪ Lead wires can vary in number and positioning
        - ◆ RA wire—placed medial to the RA appendage (arrow)
        - ◆ RV wire—tip near the RV apex (arrowhead)
        - ◆ LV wire—placed in a tributary of the coronary sinus or on the LV surface

Differential Diagnosis

- ► Other wires/tubes

Teaching Points

- ► Pacemakers have been shown to improve cardiac function, reduce the severity of symptoms, and reduce mortality and morbidity
- ► Made up of a pacemaker generator (battery pack and control unit) and lead wire(s) with electrodes contacting the endocardium or myocardium
- ► Cardiac resynchronization therapy uses three lead wires (RA-biventricular)
    - ▪ RA wire optimizes AV timing and synchronizes ventricular pacing
    - ▪ Biventricular wires promote ventricular synchrony
    - ▪ Used to treat severe CHF—increases LV size; improves EF and mitral regurgitation
- ► Pacemakers are now frequently bundled with an AICD to monitor arrhythmias and treat ventricular fibrillation and tachycardia
- ► Complications: Lead malpositioning or fracture, pacemaker twiddling (results in shortening of the leads), myocardial perforation, hemopericardium

Management

- ► When changing or removing the pacemaker, the leads are cut and left in place due to "epithelialized" leads

Further Reading

Hunter TB et al. Medical devices of the chest. *Radiographics*. 2004;24(6):1725–1746.

History

▶ A 62-year-old male with acute MI admitted to a cardiac care unit

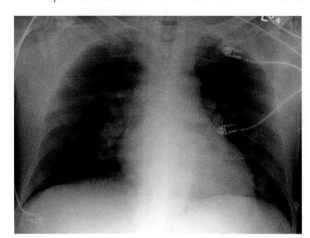

Figure 109-1   Day 1 in the cardiac care unit

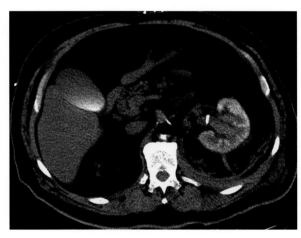

Figure 109-2   Day 5 in the cardiac care unit

Case 109 Intra-aortic Balloon Pump

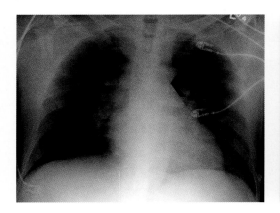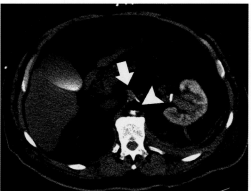

Findings

- ► CXR:
    - ▪ Access obtained from the common femoral artery
    - ▪ Proper position: Tip of the catheter projects over the aortic knob (arrow), just distal to the left subclavian artery in the descending thoracic aorta
- ► CTA: ± Associated complications, such as balloon malpositioning (arrowhead) near the origin of the superior mesenteric artery (block arrow)

Differential Diagnosis

- ► Other wires/tubes

Teaching Points

- ► Also known as the *intra-aortic counterpulsation balloon* (IACB)
- ► Made up of an inflatable 22- to 26-cm-long balloon mounted on a catheter
- ► Used to improve coronary artery perfusion and LV function in patients with cardiogenic shock or after cardiothoracic surgery
    - ▪ Balloon is inflated with carbon dioxide or helium during ventricular diastole to augment diastolic coronary artery perfusion
    - ▪ Balloon is deflated during ventricular systole, which creates negative pressure and, in turn, reduces LV afterload
    - ▪ Balloon inflation is based on either the ECG or the pressure transducer at the tip of the catheter
- ► Complications: Mesenteric ischemia (balloon malpositioning), aortic or iliac artery dissection, limb ischemia ± compartment syndrome (on the side of access), thromboembolism, infection, thrombocytopenia, balloon rupture

Management

- ► Absolute contraindication in patients with aortic regurgitation, aortic dissection, or severe aortoiliac occlusive disease

Further Readings

Hunter TB et al. Medical devices of the chest. *Radiographics.* 2004;24(6):1725–1746.
Hyson EA et al. Intraaortic counterpulsation balloon: radiographic considerations. *AJR Am J Roentgenol.* 1977;128(6):915–918.

History

▶ A 78-year-old male with ischemic cardiomyopathy awaiting heart transplantation

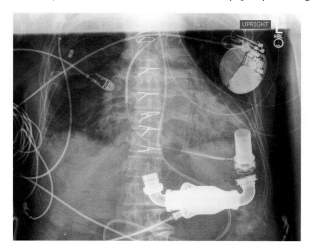

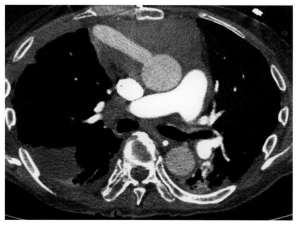

Case 110 Left Ventricular Assist Device

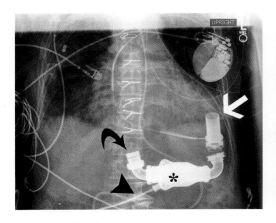 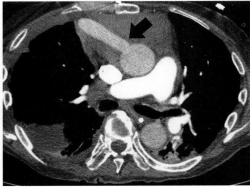

Findings

▶ CXR: Proper position: Pump (asterisk) is usually in the left upper quadrant of the abdomen with an inflow conduit (arrow) directed at the mitral valve, an outflow conduit (curved arrow) directed superiorly to the ascending aorta, and a drive line (arrowhead) originating inferiorly from the pump

▶ CTA: Assess the conduit connections to the LV apex and ascending aorta (block arrow); assess the location of the pump—within a preperitoneal pocket (preferred site), external to the abdominal viscera, or in an intra-abdominal position, ± associated complications

Differential Diagnosis

▶ LV apical aortic conduit

Teaching Points

▶ Used as a bridge to transplantation in patients with end-stage heart failure or treatment for reversible cardiogenic shock

▶ Device is implanted to enable patient ambulation

▶ Made up of a pump, inflow and outflow conduits, and a pneumatic or electrical drive line connecting the pump to an external console

  ▪ Inflow conduit is a cannula originating from the LV apex to the pump

  ▪ Outflow conduit is a Dacron graft, 12–15 cm in length, inserting into the ascending aorta, 2–3 cm distal to the aortic valve

▶ Complications Postprocedural pneumothorax or hemothorax, hemopericardium, pneumoperitoneum, infection, thromboembolism, renal failure, bowel obstruction, mechanical failure

Management

▶ Up to 2 years of durability

Further Readings

Cascade PN et al. Methods of cardiopulmonary support: a review for radiologists. *Radiographics.* 1997;17(5):1141–1155.

Knisely BL et al. Imaging of ventricular assist devices and their complications. *AJR Am J Roentgenol.* 1997;169(2):385–391.

Part 12

Postintervention/ Postoperative

History

▶ None

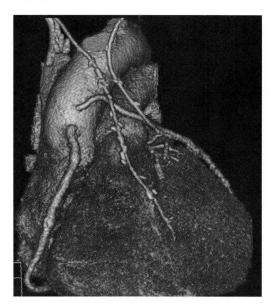

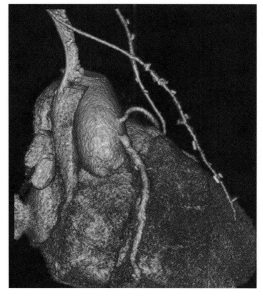

Case 111 Patent Coronary Artery Bypass Grafts

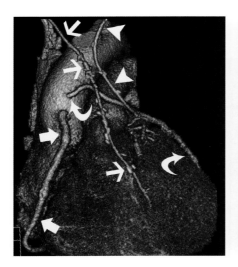
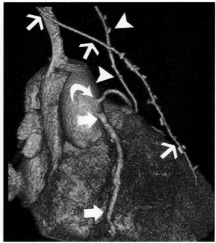

Findings

▶ CTA:
  ▪ Two types: Arterial grafts and saphenous vein grafts (block arrows)
    ◆ Arterial grafts include—in order of frequency of use—left internal mammary artery (IMA) (arrowheads), right IMA (arrows), radial artery (curved arrows), right gastroepiploic artery, inferior epigastric artery
    ◆ Arterial grafts are smaller in caliber than venous grafts
  ▪ If a graft demonstrates a homogeneous, contrast-enhanced lumen and a regular shape and border of the graft wall, it is considered patent
    ◆ Three different segments of each graft are evaluated—proximal anastomosis to the ascending aorta or origin of an in situ vessel, body of the graft, and distal anastomosis to a native coronary artery
    ◆ If the distal anastomosis is not well evaluated, the graft is considered patent as long as contrast is evident within the graft lumen

Differential Diagnosis

▶ Anomalous origin of a coronary artery
▶ Bland-White-Garland syndrome
▶ Coronary fistula
▶ Coronary artery aneurysm

Teaching Points

▶ Arterial grafts have better long-term outcomes; venous grafts are more available
▶ Complications:
  ▪ Early: Graft thrombosis (*See Case 112: Post-CABG Thrombosis*), malposition, or vasospasm, pericardial or pleural effusion, sternal infection, pulmonary embolism
  ▪ Late: Graft aneurysm

Further Reading

Frazier AA et al. Coronary artery bypass grafts: assessment with multidetector CT in the early and late postoperative settings. *Radiographics.* 2005;25(4):881–896.

History

▶ A 74-year-old male on postoperative day 9 after four-vessel CABG surgery with new onset of chest pain

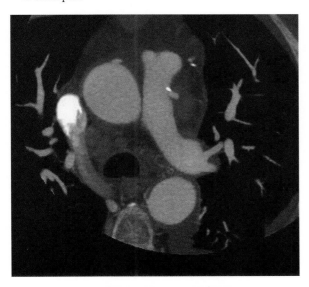

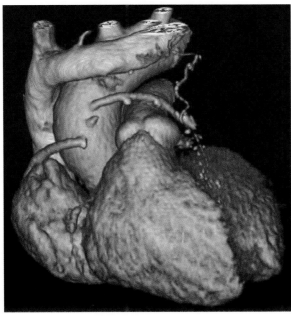

Case 112 Post-CABG Thrombosis

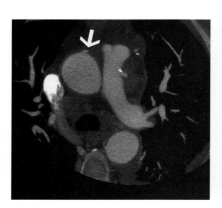 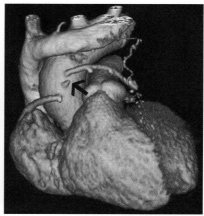

Findings

- CTA:
  - Intraluminal hypodensity without (total occlusion) and with (partial occlusion) a rim of contrast, ± calcifications, in a proximal anastomosis, body of the graft, and/or a distal anastomosis
  - Contrast filling only the most proximal part of an occluded coronary graft originating from the ascending aorta ('nubbin" sign) (arrows)
  - Part of an occluded graft may also be visible ("ghost" sign)
  - Diameter of an occluded graft can help differentiate acute (enlarged) from chronic (reduced) occlusion

Differential Diagnosis

- Coronary artery stenosis
- Post-CABG atherosclerosis

Teaching Points

- Etiology is classified into two phases
  - Early thrombosis (≤1 month after surgery):
    - Thrombosis from platelet dysfunction at the site of focal endothelial damage during surgical harvesting and anastomosis
    - Other factors, such as hypercoagulability state of the patient and high-pressure distention or stretching of the venous graft, further predispose to early graft failure
  - Late thrombosis (>1 month after surgery):
    - Atherosclerotic changes in the native coronary artery distal to distal graft anastomosis or neointimal hyperplasia in venous grafts
- Presentation: Recurrent angina, arrhythmia
- Complications: MI, heart failure, sudden death

Management

- Medical therapy (aspirin, dipyridamole, clopidogrel) to prevent thrombosis
- Endovascular (PCI + stent placement) or surgical (repeat CABG) treatment if the graft is occluded

Further Reading

Chen JJ, White CS. CT Angiography for coronary artery bypass graft surgery. *Appl Radiol.* 2008;37:10–18.

History

▸ A 76-year-old female with a history of CABG surgery and PCI with multiple stent placements presenting with new onset of chest pain

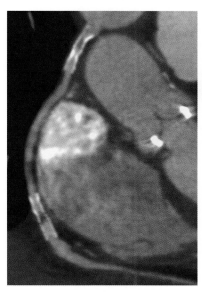

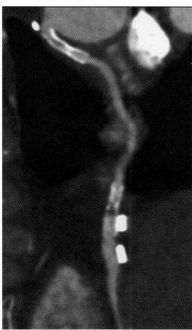

Case 113 In-Stent Restenosis

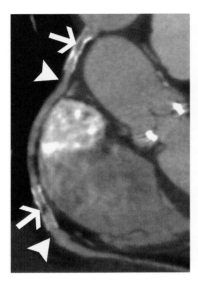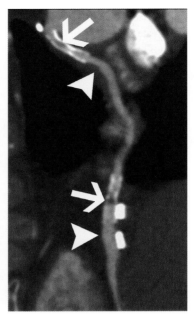

Findings

▶ CTA:
- Differentiate complete from partial in-stent occlusion
  - Complete: Stent lumen is darker than the contrast-enhanced vessel lumen proximal to the stent
  - Partial: Darker rim between the stent and the contrast-enhanced vessel lumen (arrows); >50% narrowing is considered hemodynamically significant
  - Contrast-enhanced vessel distal to the stent (arrowheads) suggests partial in-stent occlusion, although retrograde flow from collateral vessels can also give this appearance
- Stent-related beam-hardening artifacts can limit the assessment of the stent lumen and the underestimation of the in-stent intraluminal diameter

Differential Diagnosis

▶ In-stent thrombosis
▶ Coronary artery stenosis

Teaching Points

▶ Caused primarily by neointimal hyperplasia, usually a late event
▶ Risk factors: Longer stent length, smaller lumen diameter, complex lesion anatomy (e.g., an ostial or bifurcating lesion), discontinuity in lesion coverage, DM
▶ Epidemiology: 10% with a drug-eluting stent to 40% with an uncoated metallic stent
▶ Presentation: Recurrent angina
▶ Complication: MI

Management

▶ Medical therapy (aspirin, clopidogrel) to prevent stent occlusion
▶ Endovascular (PCI) or surgical (CABG) treatment if the stent is occluded

Further Reading

Pugliese F et al. Multidetector CT for visualization of coronary stents. *Radiographics.* 2006;26(3): 887–904.

History

▶ An 83-year-old female with a history of aortic stenosis

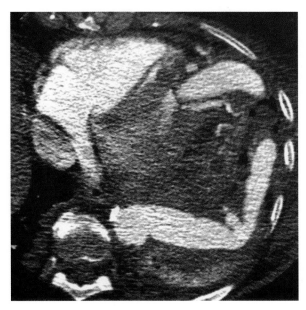

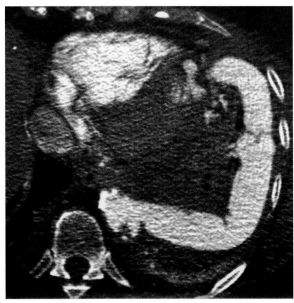

Case 114 Left Ventricular Apical Aortic Conduit

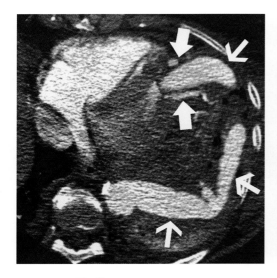 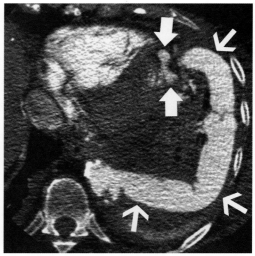

Findings

- ► CTA/MR:
  - ▪ Assess the course and angle of the implanted graft (arrows), proximal and distal anastomoses, function, and flow
  - ▪ ± Associated complications, such as a proximal anastomotic leak or pseudoaneurysm (block arrows)

Differential Diagnosis

- ► LV assist device

Teaching Points

- ► Valved graft connecting the LV apex to the descending aorta
- ► Made of Dacron, with a prosthetic valve to assist antegrade flow
- ► Used to treat critical aortic stenosis in patients with an unacceptably high risk of traditional aortic valve replacement (e.g., extensive aortic root calcification) and in patients with congenital LVOT obstruction
- ► Complications: Dysphagia, gastric erosion, anastomotic leak, periventricular pseudoaneurysm, thrombosis, arrhythmia, dysphagia, gastric erosion

Management

- ► If complicated, surgical repair may be required for treatment

Further Readings

Bickers GH et al. Gastroesophageal deformities of left ventricular-abdominal aortic conduit. *AJR Am J Roentgenol.* 1982;138(5):867–869.

Fogel MA et al. Evaluation and follow-up of patients with left ventricular apical to aortic conduits with 2D and 3D magnetic resonance imaging and Doppler echocardiography: a new look at an old operation. *Am Heart J.* 2001;141(4):630–636.

Khanna SK et al. Apico-aortic conduits in children with severe left ventricular outflow tract obstruction. *Ann Thorac Surg.* 2002;73(1):81–86.

White CS et al. Aortic valve bypass for aortic stenosis: imaging appearances on multidetector CT. *Int J Cardiovasc Imaging.* 2007;23(2):281–285.

History

- ► A 4-year-old male with a history of ASD

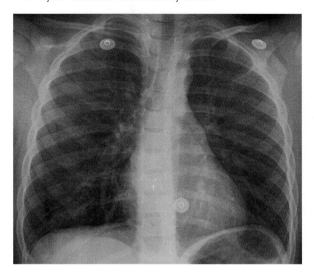

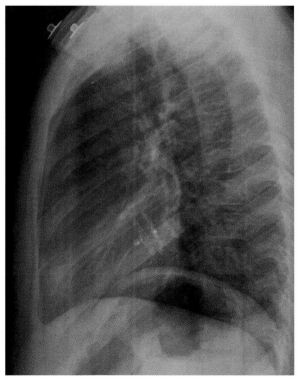

Case 115 Atrial Septal Defect Closure Device

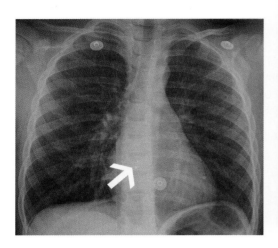

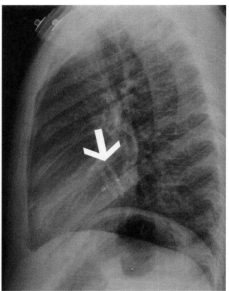

Findings

▶ CXR/CT: Assess the position and integrity of the device, ± associated complications

Differential Diagnosis

▶ VSD closure device
▶ Valvular prosthesis
▶ External lead

Teaching Points

▶ Used to permanently treat secundum ASD and PFO
▶ Made up of a basket (umbrella) or filter that expands within the ASD and straddles each side of the defect, lying flat against the atrial septum
▶ Complications: Improper placement, dislodgement, incomplete sealing of the defect, device fracture ± fragment embolism, atrial septal erosion, pericardial effusion, infection, thromboembolism

Management

▶ Short-term (at least 6 months) medical therapy (aspirin) is needed to prevent thrombus formation
▶ Prophylactic antibiotics are also recommended prior to certain medical procedures (e.g., dental surgery) to prevent endocarditis

Further Readings

Fischer G et al. Experience with transcatheter closure of secundum atrial septal defects using the Amplatzer septal occluder: a single centre study in 236 consecutive patients. *Heart.* 2003;89(2): 199–204.
Hunter TB et al. Medical devices of the chest. *Radiographics.* 2004;24(6):1725–1746.
O'Laughlin MP. Catheter closure of secundum atrial septal defects. *Tex Heart Inst J.* 1997;24(4):287–292.
Schlesinger AE et al. Transcatheter atrial septal defect occlusion devices: normal radiographic appearances and complications. *J Vasc Interv Radiol.* 1992;3(3):527–533.

Index of Cases

Index